Praise for *Li*

One of the most compassionate and encouraging books I've ever read that guides the bereaved in how to find hope and spiritual solace after loss. Filled with dozens of ideas and real-life examples, Ashley Davis Bush provides readers with "Light-shift" practices they can use to lighten grief's journey and access deeper levels of love, connection, and fulfillment beyond loss.

—Courtney Armstrong, author of *Transforming Traumatic Grief and Rethinking Trauma Treatment*

This is a beautiful book. Ashley Davis Bush shares guidance, stories and practical advice for living and growing through loss. Taking these chapters in your mind and heart will be time well spent. You will want to keep this transformational book in your life for a long time.

—Elisha Goldstein, PhD, psychologist and author of *Uncovering Happiness*

This book is a treasure, an essential guide if you've lost a loved one, whether recently or many years ago. When you are most lost, this book—like a flashlight in the darkness—will help you navigate the grief journey. Ashley Davis Bush offers practical tools along with her trademark down-to-earth, accessible wisdom.

—Diane Poole Heller, PhD, psychologist and author of *The Power of Attachment*

Brilliant! As an avid reader of and long-time fan of Ashley Davis Bush's work, her new book, Light After Loss, is another must-read . . . Whether a loss was sudden or expected, recent or long ago, readers will discover how to shift into the light of higher healing and engage in life again no matter how much darkness they may be experiencing now.

—Chelsea Hanson,
author of *The Sudden Loss Survival Guide*

Light After Loss is a beautiful compilation of spiritual comfort, psychological wisdom, and practical tools for those grieving the loss of a loved one. Ashley Davis Bush's latest work represents over thirty years of experience working with grief and is a must read and great gift to those navigating unimaginable loss.

—Erica Komisar, LCSW,
psychoanalyst and author of *Being There*
and *Chicken Little The Sky Isn't Falling*

This practical book is both guide and companion, offering warm accompaniment and the tools necessary to generate light after loss. Of the many books about grief, this one is pure gold.

—Rev. Leaf Seligman,
author of *Opening the Window* and *From the Midway*

LIGHT
AFTER
LOSS

LIGHT AFTER LOSS

A SPIRITUAL GUIDE FOR COMFORT, HOPE, AND HEALING

ASHLEY DAVIS BUSH, LICSW

VIVA
EDITIONS

Other Titles by *Ashley Davis Bush, LICSW*

Transcending Loss
Understanding the Lifelong Impact of Grief
and How to Make It Meaningful

Claim Your Inner Grown-Up
4 Essential Steps to Authentic Adulthood

Shortcuts to Inner Peace
70 Simple Paths to Everyday Serenity

75 Habits for a Happy Marriage
Marriage Advice to Recharge and Reconnect Every Day

Simple Self-Care for Therapists
Restorative Practices to Weave Through Your Workday

Hope and Healing for Transcending Loss
Daily Meditations for Those Who Are Grieving

The Little Book of Inner Peace
Simple Practices for Less Angst, More Calm

The Art and Power of Acceptance
Your Guide to Inner Peace

The Little Book of Spiritual Bliss

*With gratitude
for the angels among us*

Published in the United States by Viva Editions, an imprint of Start Midnight, LLC, 221 River Street, Ninth Floor, Hoboken, New Jersey 07030.

Printed in the United States
Cover design: Jennifer Do
Cover image: Shutterstock
Text design: Frank Wiedemann

First Edition.
10 9 8 7 6 5 4 3 2 1
Trade paper ISBN: 978-1-63228-076-3
E-book ISBN: 978-1-63228-133-3

How
Did the rose
Ever open its heart
And give to this world
All its
Beauty?
It felt the encouragement of Light
Against its Being.
Otherwise,
We all remain
Too
Frightened

—HAFIZ,
FOURTEENTH-CENTURY SUFI MYSTIC

CONTENTS

CONTENTS

LIGHT IN THE DARKNESS

The wound is the place where the Light enters you.

—RUMI

"What a beautiful bowl," I remarked. It was truly stunning. I had never seen anything like it before. I was sitting in the living room of an acquaintance, and I was mesmerized by the golden veins, the luminous web within what appeared to be a previously shattered ceramic bowl on her coffee table.

"Thank you," she replied. *"It's kintsugi."*

I later learned that kintsugi is the Japanese art form of repairing broken ceramics with "golden joinery." This method of repair was devised in the thirteenth century after the Shogun Ashikaga Yoshimatsu broke a favored tea bowl. When the initial repair proved unsatisfactory, he charged master craftsmen to come up with an artful solution. They reconstructed the bowl by joining the shards with lacquer mixed with powdered gold.

The artistic result reflected the Zen philosophy of honoring imperfections, highlighting the fractures, acknowledging beauty in brokenness. There is no attempt to disguise the damage but rather to work with it, making the fault lines glow.

Life after loss, initially, is like a broken bowl—shattered and unrecognizable—sharp edges everywhere. But *Light* after loss is the golden glue . . . gradually like a kintsugi bowl, bringing together the broken into something new: a different bowl, glowing gold. Turning your attention again and again to the divine Light in the darkness is the golden lacquer in your life. In this way, your life is formed anew, honoring the brokenness while celebrating the Light of love, compassion, faith, connection, and meaning. A spiritual approach to grief, like the art of kintsugi, creates an expanded transformation.

Stella was a sixty-five-year-old woman whose life was shattered when her twenty-one-year-old son, Robert, on a dark night, was held up at gunpoint on a Brooklyn street and then murdered. When Stella first came to see me over twenty years ago, she described a collapsed life. As a single mom, her son—her only child—had been the focus of her life. She told me, "My life is shattered now, nothing but fragments. I don't know what to do."

Over the years of her early grief, I gave Stella permission to immerse herself in her pain. With a broken heart, she began a journey of intentionally leaning into her feelings with self-compassion and surrender.

It might have been easy, and even understandable, to stay in a place of bitterness, despair, and anger. But as the years passed, Stella increasingly and purposefully shifted her attention toward the Light in her life, both within and beyond. With golden Light as the joinery, she began putting the shards of her life back together.

One way she did this was by developing new relationships with other bereaved mothers. In fact, she took upon herself a new life mission of reaching out to newly bereaved moms, with cards and simple gifts, through the national organization "The Compassionate Friends" (who offer support to families after a child dies). It became important to her to make a meaningful difference to grievers, a purpose which never would have happened if Robert hadn't died.

She still would have given anything if he had lived, of course, but through her work she celebrated him, filling the cracks of her life with gold. She was navigating the balance of engaging with the living and with the deceased. She stayed connected to Robert by talking out loud to him daily and sometimes writing letters to him, which she left at the cemetery with flowers.

Over time, she experienced an expansive healing and was able to engage with a powerful Light-shift of forgiveness. While it didn't happen easily or quickly, connection to her Higher Power allowed forgiveness of her son's murderer to enter her heart. She didn't do it on her own but found deep peace in the process. The forgiveness was for her own sake, her own inner peace.

Even now, over twenty-two years later, every year on Robert's "angelversary" (what I call the anniversary of the death day), she hosts a gathering in her backyard and invites friends, family, and other bereaved mothers to come together to honor all of their losses. In the last few years, she has added a monarch butterfly release ritual to symbolize transformation (both of their children and of themselves as survivors).

Stella still experiences regular grief bursts all these years later (which is normal), but she has learned to live with loss and love, side by side. She keeps turning her focus to the Light, again and again. She continues to grieve fully and live fully as she engages with old and new relationships. Her shattered bowl, different and yet whole, shimmers with Light.

Loss, and the associated pain—lots of pain—is the price tag for love. After a major loss, your heart shatters and life as you knew it changes irrevocably. You feel a wide range of agonizing feelings, which include sorrow, despair, guilt, regret, anger, rage, depression, and anxiety. *When will this pain end? How can I go on? I don't know how I'm going to survive this.*

If you're reading this book, chances are that you've had a loss—either recently or many years ago, either expected or unexpected. And so, you know this kind of pain that I'm talking about.

I am here to let you know that there is a path out of the darkness and back into the Light. I have been a grief counselor working with grieving individuals for over thirty years and I know there is a way. I call this way the Light-shift approach to grief.

LIGHT-SHIFTS

What is a Light-shift? Well, as its name implies, it's an intentional shift of attention toward the Light of spiritual awareness. You've probably had the experience of walking in the dark with a flashlight. The light illuminates your way, guides your steps. Similarly, Light-shifts shed Light on the dark journey of grief.

We know that what you bring to your attention matters. Instead of looking only at the trauma, the drama, the bitter pain, the searing sorrow, the injustice, the anger, the heartbreak, the depression (and there is undoubtedly plenty of all that) . . . instead, you also bring your attention to the Light.

By Light, I'm referring to the sacred, the spiritual, the divine—that which fills your heart with a feeling of peace, love, and expansiveness. Some call it Spirit, Source, God, Higher Power, Nature, Presence, Creativity, or Oneness. It is the "something more" that illuminates the good and hopeful. It is the Light that shines from all that was good in the past, all that is good even now in the present, and all the good that might come in the future.

Turning toward Light may sound impossible—or even irrelevant—when you are overcome with the darkness of grief. But it is possible, bit by bit, day by day. Doing so begins to shift your relationship with grief itself.

Here are some examples of Light-shift perspectives:

- There is more to life and death than what you can see
- Embrace the unknown
- Recognize that even when it's raining, the sun shines above the clouds
- Dawn comes after even the darkest night
- Love is stronger than death and endures eternally
- Souls reunite after death
- Bad things can lead to good
- Everything is as it should be
- The Universe has your back
- Death is simply a portal to another dimension
- Souls come to earth to learn and grow
- You will be reunited with your loved one
- There are no accidents, and we are all connected
- Choose to open your mind and welcome Mystery
- Nature is vast and beautiful, and you are a part of it

Light-shifts can be big or small, seen as a new insight or a behavior change—all of them leading to a gradual paradigm shift. Even words matter. For example, a client whom I worked with brought the urn holding her father's ashes to a shelf in her family room. His ashes were to join the ashes of her mother, her brother, and her beloved beagle. My client told me tearfully that she was bringing his ashes to the ever-growing "shelf of death" in her home. I asked her, "How would it be for you to think of it as the 'shelf of love' instead?" Later, she told me that this verbal reframe (one of many Light-shift techniques) entirely shifted her feelings for the mantle. It helped her focus on the love and not just the loss. Words can be our signposts to the Light.

Moments matter, too. When you take moments to redirect your focus, day by day, you begin to feel calm, peaceful, purposeful, loving, compassionate, wise, thoughtful, and accepting. Yes, you still live with loss, with a tender sorrow in your heart, but in choosing to turn toward the Light of Spirit, you see and experience the world from a Light-shift dimension that brings hope into your heart.

GROWING A GARDEN

Neuroscientists recognize the phenomenon that "what you focus on grows stronger." Why? Because science has shown that you strengthen neural pathways in your brain when you think or behave in the same way again and again. If you are angry on a regular basis, you will strengthen the neural pathway of anger in your brain. Practice patience? You strengthen the quality and experience of patience.

The idea is that life is like a garden—it's full of flowers but also weeds. If you shine the flashlight of attention only on the weeds, you will see weeds and feel the effects of only seeing weeds. However, if you shine the flashlight of attention on the flowers, you see more details of the flowers and your heart fills with the effects of color and beauty.

And so it is with the garden of your life, filled with grief but also with love. Both are true. While the sorrow of grief is undeniably immense and you must feel all of your feelings in order to heal, love and goodness are also there when you are ready to turn toward them.

However, some people, after a major loss, find that they never quite emerge from bitterness and depression. The good news is that it's never too late to heal, *and* there is a strategy that can help you heal: Light-shifts toward Spirit. And yes, the Light is a metaphor for spirituality in your life.

THE CORE OF SPIRITUALITY

Since this book looks at the grieving process through the lens of spirituality, it's important to understand the lens. I'm writing about an *experience*, a *feeling*, not simply a belief or an idea. And the experience or feeling that I describe is one of calm, peace, love, even joy. It's a feeling of the self falling away and a connection to "a Source both within and beyond the self."

This experience of peace and unity is common to all religions and wisdom traditions. Yet, you don't need to be religious to access it. There are many paths to the Light.

Here are some ways that you may have experienced Spirit without even realizing it:

- when you felt wonder watching the night sky or a sunset or any natural beauty.
- when you felt at peace with a beloved pet or person asleep by your side.
- when you felt calm in the woods, by a lake, by the ocean, or on top of a mountain: '*Ahhhhhhhh, peace.*'
- when you looked into the face of someone you held so dear that your heart was filled to over-flowing with love.
- when you remember a loved one who died, how much they meant to you and *still* mean to you, and you are filled with a sense of deep and enduring love.
- when you heard a piece of music (of any genre) that touched your heart and uplifted your spirit.
- when you were awestruck by a piece of art or object of beauty that created a feeling of connection to a world greater than the self.

Each of these experiences is, in their essence, a *spiritual* experience—one that connects you to something bigger than yourself. Spirituality is your home, your birthright. And it's closer than you think. The sixteenth-century French philosopher Pierre Teilhard de Chardin said, "We are not human beings having a spiritual experience. We are spiritual beings having a human experience."

While some use the word "God" to describe the source of their spirituality, for others it goes by another name, or even by no name at all. We all long to feel peace, to connect with something larger than ourselves. Don't let yourself be put off by a name. As William Shakespeare said, "A rose by any other name would smell as sweet."

These are some words to describe the indescribable:

Universe	Spirit	Lord	God
Beloved	Source	Allah	Ground of Being
Unity	Holy	Sacred	Light
Tao	Nature	Goddess	Creator
Presence	Awareness	Being	Consciousness
Essence	Life Force	Grace	Higher Power
Infinite Intelligence		Divine Energy	Great Spirit
Beauty	Chi	Benevolent One	Creative Impulse

This inner *experience* of deep peace and connectedness that speaks to something both beyond yet within each of us is the focus of this book. Whether the experience of Spirit arises in the context of your religious tradition, out of communion with nature or humanity or beauty, or out of a deep acceptance of the present moment, it is a shift to this Light dimension—this expansive reality—in which healing takes place.

A Visual of the Spiritual Grief Perspective

"You think that over time, life will begin to look the same, but it doesn't."

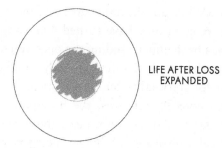

"Instead, you learn to live with it. And you *expand* around it."

RELIGIOUS INJURY OR SPIRITUAL EMPTINESS

Now maybe you are thinking to yourself, *I don't believe in Spirit* or *I have had a terrible experience with religion*. I understand. Not everyone has a positive history with religion or spirituality.

Many people have had some distasteful experiences with so-called holy moments. For some it was a judgmental or righteous insult or a shaming, punishing sense of sinfulness. For others, it might have been a platitude that minimized their pain or a traumatic childhood that cast a shadow on the idea of a heavenly father or mother. And there are some who have no connection to anything of meaning, a kind of spiritual emptiness. Either way, the spiritual baby often gets thrown out with the religious bathwater.

This book offers a completely different way of understanding the spiritual, an *expanded perspective* that opens to the unique spiritual experiences within each of us. While an uncomfortable or damaging experience with religion may have turned you away from spirituality, a fresh understanding can open you to new healing.

In this book, I offer not only "Light" as a metaphor for spirituality but also verticality. There are two dimensions in our lives, the horizontal of physicality and day-to-day circumstances (doing) as well as the vertical dimension of higher perspective and deeper understanding (being).

We can visualize Spirit as a vertical Light. a stream of energy that pours from the heavens, through you, and down into the earth. Or we can think of the verticality of a lighthouse that offers us guidance through the rough seas of life. Imagine too looking up, up to the stars above us with their vast patterns and movements, helping humans throughout history to navigate the world. The vertical is an expanded state of awareness, a more open consciousness.

If this all sounds a bit lofty, or if you're not sure about any of it, I invite you to keep your mind open. Let *"maybe"* be your new response. *Breathe. Allow. Be curious. You're on a journey of discovery.*

You might be skeptical that a vertical, Light-shift approach can ease the sharp edges of your grief, but I'm here to tell you that I have seen healing in this way again and again. Healing happens. Higher healing happens. The inspiration of witnessing healing is what has kept me working with grievers for over thirty years. I share my experiences as a hand to hold as you make your way toward the Light.

BECOMING A GRIEF COUNSELOR

How did I come to specialize in grief? In the fall of 1988, after a brief career in public relations (mostly writing press releases for allergy medications), I was burned out and longing for greater meaning in my life. After some soul searching and feeling a call to help people in emotional pain, I enrolled in social work school to become a psychotherapist. By November of that year, I was a full-time student assigned to my field placement in a community mental health center.

Flashback: It was almost 4 p.m. and the moment had come. Here I was, inexperienced and uncertain, about to greet my first ever client, about to beckon this person into my closet-sized windowless office. I advanced toward the waiting room, took a deep breath, and opened the door. Although I had little training, I was about to intimately witness the emotional struggles of another human being. I was tentative, curious, and unsure.

Although I cannot remember her name, I certainly remember her story. A middle-aged soft-spoken woman, she had come to unburden her heart. She knew that I was a resident-in-training, but she didn't hesitate to tell me her story in full and shed her many tears. Her mentally disabled sister had been killed recently by a lawn worker. Assaulted and murdered, her body had been found by my client.

This bereaved woman, my very first client, was suffering from complex grief and trauma. As she sat opposite me, she collapsed in her grief, lost and confused in an overwhelming avalanche of emotions. This emotional maelstrom might have frightened another first-time therapist, but I found within myself a natural willingness to receive and contain her feelings.

As I listened with an open heart and gave this woman permission to feel her feelings, I realized with crystal clarity, *This is exactly the kind of work that I am meant to do in this world.* In the end, I didn't find grief counseling; it found me.

Even when I ventured off into other territories in my career—working with couples, with stress management, with anxiety—I always found my way back to grievers. Perhaps it was my karmic debt in this lifetime; perhaps it was my intergenerational legacy—I just know that I was called to do it and I have tried, to the best of my ability, to answer that call.

WHAT I HAVE LEARNED

I have listened to thousands of grievers share their sorrow and confusion and devastation and regret. The core process of grieving has essentially remained the same through the years: learning to live with a tangle of overwhelming, painful emotions that come and go without warning. Grief remains as painful a process today as it has always been.

No matter the path, all grievers must feel their pain deeply. Clearly, there's no way around that. Even through the lens of spirituality, pain cannot be bypassed. In fact, it's normal for moments of pain to burst through even after many years. And yet, some people, even in spite of the pain, find a way to transform their grief. While some people get lost in the darkness, others find their way to the Light.

What makes the difference? Why would one individual be pulled to life, love, and Light but another gets lost in the darkness? Of course, many factors influence this journey, including health, history with trauma, and temperament.

But over my three decades working with grievers, I have noticed a clear pattern toward healing: spiritual grievers integrate love and compassion and a feeling of faith and connection back into their lives more easily and more quickly. They have a motivation and a willingness to shift consciousness even while holding loss in their hearts. They see loss and love as part of a larger whole and realize that they are *more* than just their grief. They are willing (either naturally or by intention) to connect to a higher awareness, to a bigger perspective.

In my therapy practice and my writing and social media posts, I work diligently to guide people toward this sense of "something more," to help them make shifts to the Light of the vertical dimension. I have seen over and over again that doing so makes all the difference on the journey. When you expand around your grief, you find a new perspective that leads to a greater sense of peace and healing.

This book is the culmination of thirty years of working with grief and loss: what I have learned and what I feel is most important to share.

This book is about helping *you* find your way on the path to higher healing.

This book is about helping *you* expand so that you'll

find relief and comfort and a personal growth journey that you never imagined.

FINDING YOUR WAY

This book will take you through the grief journey while continually holding a lamp of spirituality to light the path. In part 1, "The Journey through Pain and Suffering," chapter 1 (Shock) and chapter 2 (Help!) focus on the core of the grief work—Shock, Disorganization, and Reconstruction.

In part 2, "The Spiritual Heart of Comfort and Hope," chapters 3–6 (Love, Connection, Compassion, and Faith) look at how these vertical experiences integrate into the ongoing stage of living with loss over time known as Synthesis.

In part 3, "A Higher Healing," chapter 7 (Transcendence) looks at this sacred intentional stage of meaning-making, and how it is energized and motivated by a shift of consciousness toward the Light.

Each chapter weaves together anecdotes and case study composites (with names and details changed to protect privacy), along with the perspective of evidence-based research and wisdom traditions. Finally, each chapter concludes with five essential "Light-Shift Practices" that you can use daily.

THE LIGHT-SHIFT PRACTICES

The Light-shift Practices are simple tools and techniques designed to be a helping hand, a tender guide on your path. Use one, use all, but take them on deliberately, as you are able. They will both pave and illuminate the way. These specially curated tools will make bad better—you can't change what's happened to you, but you can find help in using these resources to shore you up.

Shifting to the Light isn't a one-time thing. Think about it: you don't just breathe once, exercise once, or eat once and then think, *Great! I'm all set now.* No, you do those things over and over again, every day, many times a day even. And you will do them every day of your life.

The same is true of Light-shifts. To be most effective, they need to be repetitive, habitual ways of living. Committing to one or more of these practices in the morning and the evening, every day, will ground you as you navigate the harsh terrain of the grief journey. Even though you might only feel a moment of Light in a day of darkness, the moments matter. They build, they expand, and they create a tipping point into higher healing.

Remember Stella from earlier in this chapter, a woman whose young adult son was murdered on a city street over twenty years ago? She still has to make Light-shifts on a daily basis to ground herself in hope and healing, lest she fall into her own self-pity. Her grief doesn't end because her love doesn't end. She focuses on the love she feels for and from her son and works to foster an ongoing connection with him. She still reaches out to newly bereaved mothers, and she still hosts her annual gathering on his angelversary.

Stella has grieved deeply and she chooses to live deeply. Forgiving the assailant freed her heart to open into compassion. She realizes every day how her awareness of "something bigger than herself" allows her to navigate a world of heights and valleys, atrocities and blessings.

Now it's your turn—your journey, your own individualized process filled with pain and at times despair. But you don't have to white knuckle your grief. You don't have to simply survive and never "get over" your loss. You can alter your relationship with grief and see it as a portal to something new. When you initiate this paradigm shift, you realize that things are not always as they seem. Grief exists only because love exists, and love can be the transformational wind beneath your wings.

In this book, I am summarizing and sharing all my years of working, living, loving, losing, watching, growing, learning, training, writing, and serving. All you have to do is read on, listen, and be curious.

And so it is that I offer this book, which I pray will guide you and light your way on your sacred journey. There will still be pain—and lots of it—but there also will be solace and comfort. Shifting to the Light of the vertical dimension reduces the severity and duration of intense painful feelings and opens the way for opportunity to arise.

You are still on this planet for a reason, and I hope that this book will help you discover why. In the meantime, don't forget that you are imprinted with rays of divine love and Light woven within your soul, now and always.

PART 1

THE JOURNEY THROUGH PAIN AND SUFFERING

As you start to walk on the way,
the way appears.

—RUMI

There once was a woman named Kisa Gotami who lived in ancient India during the same time as the Buddha. She had been devastated by grief after her only child died. Unwilling to accept his death, she carried him in her arms from neighbor to neighbor asking for medicine to bring him back to life.

One of the neighbors suggested that she go to the Buddha and see if he could help her. So, she did.

The Buddha told her to return to her village and gather mustard seeds from the households of those who had never known death. With those mustard seeds, he told her, he could create a medicine to restore her son to life.

Hopeful, the woman went from home to home, asking for mustard seeds. While the neighbors were willing to oblige, each neighbor informed her that their household had known death. Every single household, of course, had known death.

She came to realize the universality of death and that she was not alone in her sorrow. With this understanding, she was able to meet her grief with a calm acceptance. She buried her son in the forest and returned to the Buddha with the awareness that all people are touched by death.

Kisa's grief, seeded from pain, blossomed into compassion and wisdom. She became one of Buddha's disciples and went on to become the first female arahant (one who has achieved nirvana).

The Parable of the Mustard Seed serves to remind us that we are unified in our experience of death and grief. In truth, people have been grieving since the beginning of time. Currently, approximately sixty million people die every year across the world, each leaving behind a community of grieving family members and friends.

None of us is alone with this experience. Everyone, everywhere, has already or will shortly experience a deep and profound loss. It doesn't matter your nationality, socioeconomic position, country, century, age, ancestry, or education level—grief is the great equalizer.

But let's face it, our shared experience does not lessen the initial heartbreaking, soul numbing, and searingly painful blow of loss. At first, it may seem that no Light will ever again brighten your life. This section of the book talks about the painful, nonlinear, often circular journey from Shock through Disorganization and into Reconstruction.

CHAPTER 1
SHOCK

There is a candle in your heart,
ready to be kindled.
There is a void in your soul,
ready to be filled.
You feel it, don't you?

—RUMI

In a powerful documentary on loss called *Speaking Grief,* there is a scene in which every person on an urban street is wearing a blue t-shirt with white lettering that simply identifies the person they lost: "mother," "sister," "son," "granddaughter," "husband," "stepson," "cousin."

Every single one of us could wear such a t-shirt because every single one of us has lost people dear to us. Equally as universal as loss is the initial shock upon learning of a loved one's death. Shock is particularly staggering when a death is sudden, unexpected, traumatic, and/or out of the normal life cycle order. However, even when a loss occurs after a prolonged illness, or a hospice stay, when there is allegedly ample time to anticipate and prepare for the death, shock still stops you in your tracks. The weight of shock settles on your body as you shake your head in disbelief. You thought you had more time. Like grief itself, shock is universal.

"Am I going crazy?" asks one griever. "I must be going crazy," says another. "You're going to think I'm crazy," whispers a griever to me. This is a common refrain from people who have had the rug pulled out from beneath them, who have been left in the wake of death.

You may have wondered this as well. Maybe you can't find your keys; can't concentrate to read; can't remember details. Maybe you cry nonstop for hours and then laugh during a movie.

And maybe you simply cannot absorb that your loved one is gone. In your head, you get it. But in your heart, it's unthinkable. *Maybe they're just on a trip?* you think. *Maybe I can call them—oh wait, no. But how can it be true? He was here and now he's gone? Where did he go?*

After a loss, your cognitive functioning is impaired as your brain and body respond to perceived threat. As a result, it might feel like your brain is offline completely— you will be confused; foggy; disoriented. It might feel hard to make decisions or function as usual, like planning and organizing. Your brain literally is in a protective pause, unable to process and absorb all that is happening.

George is a client who experienced a devastating shock when, on Thanksgiving at noon, he heard five strong knocks on his front door. He was not greeted with a Thanksgiving pumpkin pie or good tidings from a neighbor. Instead, he was greeted with two compassionate police officers who told him that his daughter had been found dead in a hotel room that morning.

George literally dropped to the ground, unable to speak. George had been a single dad who worried chronically about his twenty-five-year-old daughter, a recovering drug addict. Apparently, after months of being clean and sober, she had lost her battle with addiction and died of a drug overdose. How can a father recover from such a loss?

We are wired to connect and when the connection is seemingly broken, we are beyond bereft.

HARD TO ABSORB

Shock can last a surprisingly long time . . . weeks for some, even months for others. In fact, if you're currently in the shock phase, you probably aren't even reading this book just yet, as it can be difficult to concentrate or absorb information. It can be difficult enough just to shower on a given day, much less read a book from beginning to end. Shock is like a protective shield to your mind and heart.

For many, shock looks like utter collapse, as it did for George. This is why some grief groups won't allow new members to join the group unless their loss occurred three or more months ago. On the one hand, I understand this requirement since most grievers are too foggy, too numb in those first three months to get much benefit out of a processing group. On the other hand, for a griever in raw pain to wait a little longer before relief can be offered can feel cruel indeed.

After Maria lost her husband of thirty-five years, she described to me not being able to believe that he was gone. She would know in her head that he had died, but then she would turn to him to tell him a story. She would look for him in the morning to see if he was already downstairs having his coffee. She even would pick up his favorite snack when she was in the grocery store, only to place it back on the shelf in tears as she realized that he wasn't at home to receive it.

One moment she would remember, with sharpness, that he was gone, but the next moment, it was as if she expected him to answer her call . . . "Joe?" She told me that she was exhausted by this back and forth, ping and pong of reality and denial, reality and denial.

It's as if the mind can't absorb all at once the enormity of this life change. Reality enters into the brain and then overflows out of the brain. It's like pouring water into a potted plant; if you pour too much, the water cannot be absorbed and simply overflows.

The griever remembers, forgets, knows but can't

believe it. *It can't be—surely that was a terrible nightmare?* But then the griever wakes up into the harsh light of day and remembers anew—*oh yes, my loved one is gone.* Life seems to be sapped of joy, of color, of hope. One day life was one way and now, the next day, everything is different.

Grieving is exhausting work, especially in the initial phase of Shock. You might find that you're physically drained, almost ill, more fatigued than you ever thought possible. You have been slammed physically, emotionally, and maybe even spiritually. You might be angry at God or simply adrift from all things vertical. If so, you're not alone in that experience.

The primary task during the shock phase is to go slow, be gentle, and take care of yourself. In the Victorian era, grievers wore a black armband for up to a year. This armband was to signify to others: "I'm grieving. Be gentle with me. I'm not my usual self." While these still exist and are even sold online, we don't typically see or wear them. It's too bad because we are just as vulnerable now as grievers were over a hundred years ago.

Think of the shock phase as having a concussion. You need to rest and cut yourself a lot of slack. You need to say "no" instead of "yes" to obligations. And you need to find comfort and self-care where you can—in flowers, in condolence notes, in blankets, in music, in hot baths, in long naps. You need tender loving care like never before. And you need support from others.

IT TAKES A VILLAGE

I once had a client whose father told him, "Don't have a funeral for me, son. It's a waste of money and I won't be there to appreciate it." What that father didn't realize is that a funeral or memorial service is less for the deceased and more for the living. Community creates a necessary web of support under the griever.

Funeral and burial rites are as old as human history. They are how we both give voice to our initial grief and honor the lives that have ended. In addition to the public acknowledgment of loss and the respectful reflection on a life, these ceremonies offer social support and companionship to the bereaved. It helps to be uplifted and held by a community when you're grieving. The flowers and cards and casseroles matter. As time goes by, the rituals of support end but the grief does not.

You can imagine the surreal experiences of virtual funerals during the Covid-19 pandemic, a loss of regular ritual in the midst of loss of life. Of course, we desperately need our rituals, which is why even Zoom services, drive-through funerals, and online memorials are better than nothing. A funeral/memorial/celebration service provides a venue for sharing memories and a net of vital communal support and love for those left behind.

Or rather, these rituals ought to provide such support. But sometimes, grievers are inadvertently hurt during a service in which pain is minimized and explanations are maximized.

LOOKING FOR ANSWERS

I have been a singer and a performer all of my life, but there is nothing quite as touching as singing at an end-of-life service. I have sung "Amazing Grace" at my grandfather's funeral, "Somewhere over the Rainbow" at my father-in-law's funeral, and "Ave Maria" at my sister-in-law's funeral. Each time was heartfelt and moving in a way that touches the soul beyond words.

But it was when I sang "Amazing Grace" at the memorial service of a neighbor that I remember encountering unintentional spiritual injury. This service was to honor and remember a thirty-seven-year-old woman who had died unexpectedly of a brain aneurysm, leaving behind her thirty-nine-year-old husband, her seven-year-old son, and her four-year-old daughter.

A memorial service for a young woman, dying in the prime of her life, leaving behind a young family feels tragic, senseless. During the reception, I heard a well-meaning friend speaking to the widower. He began to talk about God s will and concluded his remarks with "God must have needed another angel in heaven."

I looked over at the young widower, clearly uncon-soled—in fact, even angered—by his friend's words. Later, I chatted with the widower privately. He knew that I was a therapist, and he looked at me beseechingly, "Do you think this was God's will?" I was a bit shocked by his forthright question. In classic therapist form, I turned the question around, "Well, um, do *you*?"

His eyes were rimmed red. "Honestly," he offered,

"I don't see why God would need any more angels—he has enough. I needed a wife and my children needed their mother."

I answered softly, "Of course." There really were no explanations, no pithy rationales. So, I simply gave him a hug.

No one means to be unkind at a funeral, certainly. People simply don't know what to say when faced with vast pain and overwhelming loss. In fact, it's fair to say simply that "I don't know what to say," or "I can't imagine how you're feeling," or "Nothing about this makes sense."

We want answers, but we don't have answers. As a result, people say all sorts of things at funerals that unintentionally create a spiritual injury—"It was her time," "God needed her more," "Trust in the Lord." Maybe these comments are meant to provide solace, and maybe for some, they do. However, at the funeral, when all is so sharp and jagged—the best thing is to show up with fewer words and more nonverbal support, like a hug or a shared tear. An authentic desire to be present and express your kindred sorrow is itself a kind of spiritual comfort.

LOOKING FOR LIGHT

So how do you look for Light when everything is so dark and foggy? Well, for those with an already estab-lished spiritual or religious life, there can be immediate comfort in that. I have known many grievers to quickly turn to prayer, meditation, and religious services/community for support.

Whether from a church, ashram, synagogue, or bowling league, community is Light. George, for example, whose daughter overdosed on Thanksgiving Day, was blown away when his bowling league created a dinner "tree" for him so that he didn't have to cook any dinners for a month. George felt held even as his heart was shattered. His bowling group became a vehicle for Light, offering him consolation without fixes. There were no glossy spins, just the nourishing, loving presence of a Light-filled community. And in this, the seeds of healing were planted.

If you don't have a ready-made community or faith base, the internet provides a literal web of support in a variety of grief-related chat rooms, interactive community pages, and online support groups. Virtual support is a Light resource of compassion and connection that our ancestors could have never even imagined.

Even with Light coming from a variety of places, the heavy darkness of initial Shock and early grief can be like a lead blanket over your heart and even your body. But over time, you will feel moments when the weight lifts, bit by bit. To aid the healing journey, I suggest that you look upward to the sky, as often as you can, day or night. Look up and notice the changing sky, the clouds, the colors. Notice the stars and the waxing moon. Notice that there is more, a vast universe, a bigger picture. You are part of it, and loss is part of it as well.

Shock collapses us inward, which is normal, but allow yourself to remember that there is an expanded universe, even in the midst of calamity.

For most people, after the funeral/memorial service, after the casseroles and cards, after the fog, after others have gone back to their busy lives, they are left alone. You might be feeling alone . . . very alone. Now, the real grief work begins.

Shock turns out to be the tip of the iceberg of the grief journey. I'm reminded of the classic line delivered by Bette Davis in the 1950 Hollywood film *All About Eve*: "Fasten your seat belts, it's going to be a bumpy night."

Yes, you're on an inescapable journey, but the helpful news is that there is medicine for the soul. Assistance, coping strategies, and support are here and available and we're going to be exploring them together. You don't have to go into the bumpy night alone because you are surrounded by the energy of your loved one, the Spirit of "something more," and the solidarity of millions of grievers who have been on the same journey throughout all of human history.

LIGHT-SHIFT PRACTICES

1—Sacred Music

Music throughout the ages has often been associated with spiritual soothing and upliftment. Music soothes the dying, comforts Alzheimer's patients, and narrates the moods across our life spans. Music lifts us out of ourselves and connects us to something more. It's like a portal to the Light that resides within and beyond us.

The Practice

Listen intentionally to some sacred music. You may already have some favorites, or you can experiment with different genres: gospel music, contemporary country, Christian, Buddhist chants, Indian kirtans, Gregorian chants, Native American flute music, Western sacred choral masses and requiems (such as Mozart, Bach, or Verdi). While many types of music can be calming or uplifting, I suggest that you try specifically sacred music, written by people throughout the ages who have crafted music to touch the Divine. Notice how it moves you.

However, all music has the potential to awaken your inner Light and direct you to the Divine. So, if traditional sacred music doesn't move or touch you, then listen to any music that feels sacred, that is, that brings you to an expansive, uplifted, or deep place.

2–TLC Basket

The experience of shock, whether it's from trauma or grief, requires what is known as Psychological First Aid. Psychological First Aid was devised in 2006 by the National Center for Post-Traumatic Stress Disorder in order to reduce the occurrence of PTSD. Research had shown that debriefing—discussing the trauma immediately after the fact—was traumatizing in itself. Instead, for fostering short and long-term adaptive functioning, it was better to focus immediately on stabilization, safety, and comfort.

Two of the key components of Psychological First Aid are creating a sense of safety and creating a sense of calm. A self-soothing basket that assembles something for each of your senses acts on this same principle.

The Practice

Assemble in a basket or other container items that make you feel emotionally safe, items that make you feel calm. Once assembled, spend some time with your basket each day, for at least ten minutes at a time, or as needed. Go through its contents, one at a time, mindfully aware, as an intentional way to provide relief for your weary mind, body, and soul.

Use the 5 senses as your guide:

Touch: Choose something soft and/or weighted. A weighted blanket has been connected with reducing anxiety. A soft flannel shirt could also be comforting—

especially if it was worn by your loved one. I've known many grieving individuals to have a seamstress take old shirts of their beloved and craft them into either a teddy bear, a pillow, or a quilt. This has the added comfort of being soft and cozy but also being a direct connection to your loved one.

You might consider a teddy bear or stuffed animal to cuddle. Most adults don't have teddy bears to hold in their own dark nights of the soul, but they can be surprisingly comforting.

Wrap yourself and touch each treasured item. What do your fingers sense with regard to texture? How does it feel to touch this?

Taste: Peppermint, chamomile, or your favorite tea or beverage. Or pick a candy, mint, or nut. Close your eyes and savor the flavor. What stands out to you?

Smell: Lilac or citrus, balsam fir, menthol or incense, a candle, spray, mister, atomizer. Inhale the scent—what feeling do you associate with it? How does it make you feel right now?

You could also choose to smell a jar of peanut butter or ground coffee, something that is pleasing to you.

Sound: A bell, chime, or singing bowl. Or perhaps a drum. Take a moment to create the sound. Listen to the sound waves as they dissipate. Notice the effect on your nervous system.

Sight: An object that is special to you. It can be a memento or something that belonged to your loved one. It can also be an object from nature, such as a shell or stone which you can both see and touch. Or you can also include a crystal or stone such as rose quartz or lapis lazuli. You could add a few items to be visually appealing—something brightly colored and something else with a neutral palette.

Take a moment to look at each item, examining the smallest details. Stop. Look longer. Are there memories associated with this item? How do you experience the color? Imagine its journey to get to the palm of your hand.

3—A Thousand Words

They say that a picture is worth a thousand words. Photographs can be a contemplative balm, a window into beauty. Fortunately, in our technological world, we can access gorgeous photos with the click of a button. When you take photographs on as a means of self-care, you choose photographs that will either lift your spirits or calm your soul.

Consider sacred architecture and natural wonders to stir your soul and turn you toward the Divine. Gaze and be amazed.

The Practice
Search the internet (or books) for images that inspire awe and wonder. Spend several minutes with a photograph

and notice how your mind and body react. You might even want to frame a photo that is especially powerful for you, or save it on your phone or computer's screensaver. Slow down and be with the image, absorbing its impact on you.

Here are some categories to search:

Nature photos	Landscapes
Wild animals	Ancient forests
Ocean waves	Lakes
Mountaintops	Butterflies
Flowers	Seasons
Rainforests	Milky Way
Sanctuaries	Ashrams
Cathedrals	Stained glass windows
Temples	Synagogues
Mosques	Church spires
Space—Search photos from the Hubble Telescope Station or NASA's "Out of This World" series	

4—The Calm Breath

The 4-7-8 breath is an ancient yogic breath known to recalibrate the nervous system. With regular use, many people experience greater clarity and reduced anxiety. When you're experiencing the shock of grief, you might feel numb, dazed, even out of your body. Your breath can help calm you, orient you to the now, and bring you back into your body.

The Practice
Breathe in through your nose for the count of 4. Hold your breath for the count of 7. Exhale through your mouth (as if you're blowing out through a straw) for the count of 8. Repeat this cycle two more times.

5—That's a Wrap
You have a self-soothing strategy right at your fingertips (and your palms). Grief is a form of emotional trauma, and the following technique is used to soothe and calm trauma victims.

The Practice
Wrap your right hand across your forehead and wrap your left hand across the back of your head. Breathe low and slow. Then, keep your right hand across your forehead and place your left hand on the upper chest. Breathe low and slow. Notice how your body starts to settle and shift. Finally, keep your left hand on the upper chest and bring your right hand off of your forehead and place it on your belly. Breathe deeply, letting your belly expand with each breath.

CHAPTER 2
HELP!

If the Light is in your heart,
you will find your way home.

—RUMI

I stood at the podium looking out over a sea of sad faces. Actually, sad is too inadequate a word. Crushed. Lifeless. Shattered. Each person wore a badge with the face of a deceased young person—their son or daughter who had died within the last year. This was a somber occasion to honor loss, yet the mission of this service was also to celebrate love and life.

I was the speaker at this children hospital's annual service for the families of patients who had died in the past year. The burden of bereaved parents outliving their children, an unexpected out-of-life-cycle loss, shocks our sensibilities. Bereaved parents have a glazed look.

I opened my talk with the image of a star dying in the Universe. "When a star dies," I said, "its light continues to shine for millions of years. And so, it is with your children. Their Light shines upon you and out from within you. Their Light continues to shine brightly."

I went on to normalize their experience, validate their ongoing pain, offer suggestions for self-compassion, and remind them of what they already knew—that they, like all grievers, were changed forever.

But does this mean that a person is unable to heal? No. Does it mean that a person cannot move forward? No. In the same way that each of us is touched irrevocably by love, each of us is touched irrevocably by loss. Every griever is changed, and to pretend otherwise is a lie. But healing happens within the change.

After my talk and a candle lighting ceremony to honor each of the children who had died, a woman came up to me with tears in her eyes. She said, "What you said is true. I lost a baby, stillborn, ten years ago and that little girl has always been in my heart. And now, I've lost another child, and well . . . it's almost unbearable. I know the pain that's coming . . . I know I have to go through it . . . and I know that there's no other way."

I teared up with her as she reached for my hand. She continued, "I like to think of them as my stars—two of them—shining down on me. And I know that it's my job to keep their Light shining through me."

* * *

Grief is not a pathology. It's a normal response to the universal experience of losing a loved one. Yes, after the funeral or memorial service, the burial or cremation, the casseroles and cards, the time off from work—other people go back to their own lives and you are left with your grief. Now the grief work truly begins. The problem, however, is twofold: (1) There will be people in your life who cannot tolerate your pain and will want you to return to your old self (you can't), and (2) You may feel that you cannot tolerate your own pain and want to avoid it (that's natural).

Interestingly—if we have a terrible pain in our shoulder, we will go see a doctor. Maybe we'll get anti-inflammatory medication. Maybe we'll need physical therapy or sonogram treatment. Or maybe we will be diagnosed with a torn rotator cuff and we'll need surgery. We search for a solution to *stop the pain*.

If the pain in our bodies can be stopped, why can't the pain in our hearts, in our minds, in our emotional centers? The reality, however, is that emotional pain cannot be quickly stopped. It can heal, but paradoxically the way to heal emotional pain is to actually *feel* it. Head on. Over and over.

UNDERSTANDING THE JOURNEY

Grief has many faces—it can look like Elizabeth Kubler Ross's famous model of dying: denial, anger, bargaining, depression, and acceptance. But the natural process is, of course, not that linear. Grief can also look like regret, resentment, guilt, helplessness, sorrow, despair, and hopelessness. Grief is a shape-shifter and its many manifestations sneak up on you, often without warning.

Part of the confusion and disorientation of grief is that it is *not* a linear journey. You don't simply progress, heal, evolve, and then reach transformation. You don't move from caterpillar to chrysalis to butterfly. It's more like caterpillar, chrysalis, back to caterpillar to chrysalis to butterfly and then back to chrysalis. You might think that the highs and lows, the back and forth, the round and round, the better then worse, the roller-coaster dizzying repetition of it all means that you're doing it wrong. But guess what? That's grief and it *is* a crazy ride.

I frame the grief journey with the following broad "phases": Shock, Disorganization, Reconstruction, Synthesis, Transcendence. As discussed, *Shock* is when the loss first occurs and you can't quite take it all in. Grievers going through Shock tend to think that they're going crazy. The darkness, confusion, and over-whelming numbness can be quite intense.

After the darkness lifts, you're left with *Disorganization*, the heart of grief. In this phase, which can last several years, grief is in the foreground of your life. You start to unpack all of the losses and see how they affect you physically, emotionally, and spiritually. It's not just your loved one who is gone—there are secondary losses as well. Relationships change and are lost as a result of the death. It might be the couple you used to socialize with who leave you, a widow, behind. Or maybe it's your friends from your child's school who leave you, a bereaved parent, behind. It could be long-term friends or family who cannot tolerate your pain. You're probably surprised by who shows up and who disappears.

Adding insult to injury, friends might not be your only secondary losses. You may have to move (losing a home, a community); you might lose your job (being unable to focus or produce); you might have financial strains. You realize that you've lost a future as well—watching your child grow up, spending retirement with your spouse. Loss leads to more loss. All of this hurts immensely, as a cascade of feelings washes over you, from depression, despair, sorrow, longing, and frustration to anger, guilt, and anxiety.

If Disorganization was a season, it would be winter—not a bright snowy blue-sky sort of winter day, but instead a bone chilling slate gray winter day. As I used to think during the frigid months of my twenty-three years living in New Hampshire, *You can't make it be summer when you're in the bleak mid-winter.* Wishing won't make it so. So, you might as well hunker down with a wool sweater and some tea and settle in by the fire.

It can seem like Light is nowhere to be found. You are basically staring at the shards of your shattered bowl of life, and it may feel like repair is impossible. Yet, somehow, from the tiniest pinpricks of Light a metamorphosis begins to take place.

As you slowly move into the phase of *Reconstruction*, grief becomes the backdrop of your life. You still toggle between the Disorganization and the Reconstruction experiences, but there is more energy to reinvest, and glimpses of Light become ever more frequent. Now you start to adjust to a new world; you venture slowly into gluing the pieces of the bowl of life back together again. You decide what fits, what is discarded. You decide who you want to be and how. You reengage with the living, with Spirit, and start to choose life again.

Synthesis is living with loss over time, holding love and loss in your heart side-by-side, while staying connected to your loved one. It means having grief "bursts" from time to time in which grief feels raw and sharp, even after many years. It means remembering, living, moving forward, while also continuing to miss your loved one. And *Transcendence*, which we'll be discussing later in the book, is when you brush the cracks of the broken bowl of your life with gold. You create purpose and see beauty in the brokenness. Kintsugi.

GRIEVING FULLY, LIVING FULLY, CHOOSING THE LIGHT

There is simply nothing like the overwhelming, ongoing emotional journey that is *grief*. It is the hardest emotional work that exists. And while it may be universal, it is wildly misunderstood. People often think that it's a short process, a time-limited process, and that pain should be avoided or at least minimized.

I spend a lot of time normalizing and validating the roller-coaster of grief. Yes, grief feels like waves, like downpours, like a spiral, like a confusing enemy. And it can change from day to day. It's normal to limit your grief to manageable "doses"—you might cry in the shower, cry while driving your car, then show up for work and act normal, then come home and spend the night in bed with tissues.

Certain factors will affect your ongoing grief: your relationship to your loved one, your culture, whether or not they were your primary attachment figure, the manner of death (sudden or expected), your age, the age of your loved one, your prior history with loss and trauma, your mental and physical health, your personality, your religious history, your spiritual inclination, and your social support network.

Grieving—with all of the darkness—is agonizing and exhausting, so it makes sense that you might try to avoid it. Our culture doesn't embrace grief or make space for conversations about loss. It's tempting, in fact, to distract yourself from overwhelming emotion—

drinking, drugging, shopping, eating, working, playing video games, gambling, watching screens. We want the pain to stop. We want the phase of Disorganization to be short and sweet. We want the five days of paid bereavement leave (offered by many companies) to wrap it all up.

Yet we have to function in a real world, so it can feel like there's no time to grieve. We have to pay the rent or the mortgage, do the grocery shopping, pay the bills, feed the children, clean the house, mow the lawn. The rest of the world goes on as if nothing has changed, and so we must pick up and carry on.

There's the conundrum: you feel as if you can't go on, but you must go on. And so you do, putting one foot in front of the other, like walking through mud. Grieving imposes itself on you: you face it and take a break, you lean into it and take a break. Until one day, it becomes a little bit easier to laugh, a little bit easier to remember with more love and less pain. You start to look forward and not just backward. You step into your future one "now" at a time.

TIME AND HEALING

While grief can feel unbearable at times, we are also wired for resilience. Every day offers moments to shift to the Light, to be lifted by the "something more" of Spirit. I often ask the people I'm working with to tell me about other times in their lives when they overcame difficult circumstances. While we all have loss stories, we also have survival stories.

They say that "Time heals all wounds," but I'm here to tell you that time alone will simply be time passing. It's how you use the time that heals. Part of your task is to hold on for the bumpy ride. Lean into your experience. When you allow yourself to fully embody Shock and Disorganization, you will heal. Yes, there is effort along with courage and curiosity as you allow the physical, emotional, and spiritual tasks of grieving to unfold.

In other words, the pain has a purpose. Feeling, expressing, digesting, and metabolizing the complex feelings encompassed by "grief" is a necessary process for healing. Giving yourself permission to feel your feelings is, in fact, what allows you to heal over time. It will propel you into the future and open you to the Light all around. Although it feels counterintuitive, your task is to lean into the pain.

People do this in different ways, of course. We each have our own style with processing pain. You might do this publicly or privately, loudly or quietly. Some people will tell every stranger they meet about their loss. Others will talk with dear friends about how life has changed and how hard it is. Others will get online and talk to strangers who understand. Some will cry alone while others cry in grief groups. Even tears themselves are healing as they rid the body of toxins and waste products while releasing endorphins.

Some people naturally shift to the Light by

expressing their feelings through art, music, ritual, or prayer. Others will find expression with a journal or by hammering wood. Some will talk about how their loved one died, and others will talk about how their loved one lived. Healing happens by acknowledging and moving the energy, keeping the emotions in motion.

If you try to cheat the process by leapfrogging right over the hard parts, the unacknowledged, unfelt, and unexpressed pain has a way of catching up with you. Unexpressed grief, showing up as a physical illness, bitterness, anxiety, depression, anger, or relationship stress, will find its way into your life.

Of course, sometimes you simply cannot allow yourself to break down. Maybe you're in a time in your life when you don't have the luxury to feel your feelings, you have to soldier on. The good news is that it's never too late to immerse yourself in raw feeling, even if many years have passed. Grief waits for you.

As a grief counselor, working with a griever would be sad work indeed if I didn't know that love, hope, and healing are the fruits of the grief work.

Grief is ultimately a *healing* process. Because I know this, I am able to guide grievers into the pain. It is the quickest path to healing. In this way, grieving is a journey. It's a journey that will take you to places of new growth and unexpected vistas, but first you're going to spend some time in the dark forest.

As you find yourself confused and alone in this

gloomy forest of early grief, I invite you to stop and breathe. You might notice Light filtering through the trees. And you might hear a bird or see a friendly frog on the path. Yes, it will be dark at times, but there's a lamp and an extra flashlight and a backpack of useful tools, and even an air mattress for when you're tired— oh, and here are some protein bars and reading materials to sustain you on the journey. In other words, it's a hard journey, yes, but there are people and tools to assist with the coping, some tried and true strategies to ease the way, guide your path, and facilitate the healing so you can find yourself, eventually, out of the forest and in the midst of a Light-filled wildflower meadow.

PAIN VERSUS SUFFERING

> Pain is inevitable in this life.
> Suffering is optional.
> Higher Healing is possible.

The pain of grief is inevitable and necessary. We don't like pain, but the pain has a purpose: to metabolize and heal the grief. I was recently shocked when a beloved principal of a nearby school was killed in a car accident at the end of the school year. One of the parents called me for advice, asking, "Should I plan activities all summer to distract the kids from their sadness?" No. Teach them that it is healthy to turn toward the pain, to notice the hurt, to share the sadness—don't teach them the fine art of distraction and numbing.

Pain is challenging at times, but it is still different from suffering. Suffering is caused by pain *plus* resistance. When you can't absorb or accept what has happened, you may spend a lot of time thinking things like, *This shouldn't have happened. If I had done things differently, it wouldn't have happened. I'm going to make someone pay for this. I can't accept that this happened. This cannot be. No!!!*

Some resistance, and therefore some suffering, is not unusual. In fact, it is a normal part of the initial stage of shock and denial. However, chronic resistance leads to getting stuck in suffering. Over time, this leads only to more suffering.

When you surrender the resistance, the feeling of *No, this shouldn't have happened; it was supposed to be different*, then you are free to move forward on the journey.

In my book, *The Art and Power of Acceptance*, I unpack what acceptance means and doesn't mean. Acceptance doesn't mean liking what happened, nor does it mean giving up. Active acceptance simply means a graceful flow with truth. The three-pronged process I describe in that book includes resistance, alignment, and possibility.

Resistance, applied to grief, is the feeling of *No, this can't be*. Alignment is when you flow with what is actually happening, when the reality moves from your head to your heart. The key ingredient to shifting from "No" to "Yes" is self-compassion. In that book, I teach the ACT practice of self-compassion (Acknowledge your suffering, Connect to others who have felt what you feel, Talk kindly to yourself). We'll be talking more about this practice in chapter 5 on Compassion. Suffice it to say that when you align with your experience just as it is, even the feeling of resistance, you create a gentle energy of support that allows things to eventually shift from the "No" to the "Yes."

Suffering (aka resistance) keeps you stuck. Acceptance, with pain, initiates healing.

BEARING THE UNBEARABLE

I walked into the hotel conference room to set up my PowerPoint presentation. I was the weekend speaker for a group of about fifty women, widows of all ages, who were gathering for their annual retreat.

As women started assembling, hugging each other and chatting, I watched them connect and comfort each other. The idea of "tend and befriend" came to my mind. The retreat organizers had put together gift bags which included lavender sprays, candles, mints, journals, poem magnets, tissues, and a black armband to wear through the weekend.

Suddenly, the idea of a formal presentation seemed out of place—too cold, too distant. I wanted to connect with these women and help them make bad better . . .

because that's the way to make the unbearable bearable. I jettisoned the PowerPoint slides and instead spoke from my heart, engaging the women with eye contact, smiles, laughter, and even tears.

Grief is a challenging but necessary process, and we want to explore all of the ways to make it more bearable. The three most important paths to managing grief are connection, expression, and self-care.

Connect with others—The groups that I helped facilitate that weekend were transformational. Women sharing with other women who understood about their feelings, about their challenges, about their kids and families and memories. This connection created a healing, magical atmosphere. It was a spiritual experience, one of grievers connecting with something bigger than themselves through their shared vocabulary and common emotional experiences.

Express your feelings—These women experienced how expressing their feelings through art, music, journaling, poetry, and photography had a transmuting effect on their grief. That which was so heart-breaking opened to love and creative spirit in a way that brought them all closer to their deceased loved ones and to each other as a community.

Self-care soothes the heart—Self-care is different for different people and at different times. One day you might need a nap, while another day you would benefit from a yoga class. During this retreat, options abounded for quiet time, massages, meditations, reiki sessions, a jazz concert, art activities, and psychic readings. I watched and encouraged these women to witness and care for themselves and each other with love and openness.

A community of tolerance, compassion, and comfort—along with many tears—made a heartfelt weekend experience that was restorative for all of us.

AS TIME GOES BY

As you're starting to realize, grief is not logical or predictable. You don't simply finish one phase and start the next. You thought you had gone through most of it and suddenly it's back again. You can think of grief like a spiral—you are going around and around, but each time you come back to the starting point you are at a higher or a deeper level.

Another helpful metaphor is to think of grief like the ocean. You stand on the shore and experience wave upon wave of grief's force. Many times, the waves come in huge surges, twenty-foot-high tidal waves, tsunamis that crash you to your knees and sweep you away. And then, other times, the waves are gentler and simply lap over your toes.

Over time, as you move up the beach, the waves continue, but they do so with more space between the waves and with less intensity. And then, you simply realize that you're spending more time on higher ground, living again, with less time battered by the waves. Grief becomes the subtle backdrop, the distant sound of the surf.

MOVING FORWARD

As you get through the year of firsts without your loved one on planet Earth, you dip in and out of Disorganization and Reconstruction, forest and clearing, clearing and back to the forest. You face the holidays, the birthdays, the anniversaries, the seasons, and every first that you never wanted to face.

Some say that the second year is even harder than the first year. Why? Because the reality of life without your loved one's presence just keeps getting more and more real. It's possible that you thought everything would be better after the first year, so when it's not, it's a sad surprise.

On top of all this grief, people are expecting you to get back to your old self, not realizing that everything has changed for you. So, you keep going day by day. They want you to "move on" (without your grief), when really you need to "move forward" (with it).

I remember Rob, a widower who told me that he absolutely could not get through the first Christmas. He told me over and over again, "I don't know how I'm going to get through this." I would tell him, "You're going to take it one day at a time, one hour at a time, and one minute at a time. And you're going to gather your resources so you know you're not alone."

Even though he felt very alone, he was open to shifting his attention to some Light in his life. One winter, I learned that he loved the sounds of birds but was sad that bird songs were absent during the cold New England winter. So, I suggested a birdsong app on his phone that he could listen to as a kind of meditation every day.

Before he knew it, it was spring, and he was able to hear real life birdsongs again. Rob told me, "I think the birds called me back into my life. Technology definitely worked in my favor. Somehow, I'm still here."

Over the next six months, Light-shifts became more frequent for Rob. He began spending more time involved with his life and less time crying. I reminded him over and over that he could move forward *with* his wife in his heart and that he never had to leave her behind.

I knew he was turning a corner when he was able to enjoy photographs of his wife. In the acute phase of grief, photographs can feel like a knife in your heart. They highlight absence and may create a flood of feelings. For Rob, he couldn't look at photos of his wife at all, initially. However, over time, photographs became a portal to the Light, treasured gifts reminding him of happier times.

It's a milestone when a griever can start to take pleasure out of looking at photographs, even if they also cause some pain. A bittersweet, sorrow-joy reaction begins to take place. And for Rob, that's exactly what happened.

I continued to work with Rob for several more years. It was only in the third year of our work together when Rob reported that he could "see life in full color again." In his first two years of grieving, Light in its full spectrum came only in bursts amidst the backdrop of gray. But in the summer of our third year of work, he said, "My God. The greens are so green this year. The flowers are so colorful." And the birds were so full of song.

Some people see in full color again within a year . . . for others, it takes more than three years. Everyone is different, just as every love relationship is different. But as you do the work, as you shift again and again toward the Light, a change occurs and brings renewed energy.

For Rob, another big shift occurred, also in his third year. Rob came into our session somehow lighter than I'd seen him before. He told me he was ready to investigate online dating. He wasn't in a rush, but he felt that sharing his life with someone was more comfortable for him than living alone. He knew that he could obviously never replace his beloved, but he was ready to embrace life again.

At some point—different for each person—there is more energy for life. You still have grief bursts from time to time, but there is a different quality to your day-to-day living. You are living more in Reconstruction rather than Disorganization, more in the wildflower meadow and less in the forest. And one day, who knows, you might find yourself having a picnic surrounded by butterflies.

THE ROLE OF SPIRITUALITY

Where does spirituality fit into the picture of grieving, feeling, and healing? For some, spirituality becomes an immediate resource, a reliable anchor. This could manifest as prayer, meditation, lighting candles in a church, talking to a Higher Power, spending time in nature, listening to sacred music, putting offerings at an altar, reading spiritual texts or scripture, attending spiritual services or talking with spiritual friends, devising spiritual rituals, giving to others, volunteer work, creative inspiration, or holding mala beads/prayer beads/rosary beads. While active spirituality doesn't take away your painful feelings, it makes them easier to bear and creates context for healing.

For some, it might be that a spiritual journey unfolds initially not with comfort but with anger. I have heard hundreds of grievers first feel extremely angry with a Higher Power—"How could the Divine allow my loved one to suffer?" "Why didn't God prevent her death?" "Where was 'a Loving Universe' in the hospital?" A person needs to start where they are. All journeys begin in one place and end in another. I encourage grievers to honor their anger.

While anger and strong emotions are all part of a natural process, if one holds open the possibility of a spiritual faith—even just a sliver of "maybe"—the Light has room to dawn. Think of the image of a bow and arrow. Before the arrow shoots forward, you first have to pull it backward. With spirituality and grief, you may find that you go backward before you go forward. Let that be the path, and don't judge the journey. Just keep the "maybe" in your back pocket.

Leanne was a client of mine who came to see me as her husband was dying. He had a terminal, inoperable brain tumor. I knew that Leanne was a religious woman whose faith had often been a source of comfort to her. We met during the difficult final hospice days and reflected on what the Virgin Mary had gone through: an agonizing process of watching a beloved person in her life (Jesus) suffer and die.

Leanne told me that after our discussion, she was open to feeling Mary's presence with her as she sat by her husband's bedside, held his hand, and whispered to him that she would be all right and that he had permission to go. She felt that Mary's presence gave her a strength and a comfort that she hadn't had before. A spiritual connection helps us do what we cannot do when we feel alone.

LIGHT-SHIFTING

Grief cracks you open. Shatters you. At times, it's simply an effort to get through your day. But healing is possible and invitations for higher healing abound.

Annie was a forty-six-year-old woman who had the blessed honor of holding her husband, Michael as he was dying. She had nursed him through his colon cancer and was bracing for his exit. As she watched him die, she began to talk to Mother Earth, asking for support. She wasn't asking for a cure or a different outcome, simply for peace and comfort for her husband.

As Annie described his death to me, she shared that, "It was like Mother Earth really was with us. I mean, nature is all about seasons, changes, recycling. I kept thinking of a tree dropping its leaves. I have always been comforted by the essence of nature and creation. When I shifted my attention to the Light of my faith, when I tapped into that force, I was able to be at peace as I watched my husband exit his body and slip away to his next season."

Annie wasn't angry. Her understanding of Spirit (through nature) brought her consolation. Annie spent the next years grieving and acknowledging her feelings, but she was also grateful for the love and life that she had had with Michael. As she spent more time in the meadow (Reconstruction) and less time in the forest (Disorganization), she could more and more frequently glimpse love amidst the rubble of loss. For her, she really came to intimately understand the concept of bittersweet: bitter in the sense of her ongoing sorrow, but sweet in her simultaneous ongoing gratitude.

She told me she felt herself expanding, relaxing, and embracing Mother Nature so that she felt lighter and lighter. Annie still missed Michael every day, but she was able to see his death as an integral part of nature's cycles.

The experience of spirituality is so much more than a belief in a Higher Power. It's a sense of something more, that this life experience is expansive and deep, beyond the bounds of your physical body and mind. That's why connecting to nature is so often a spiritual experience. And sometimes connecting to others is how you go vertical.

Joey had a strong distaste for religion. He was angry with God after his baby was stillborn and bristled at even the idea of spirituality. But shortly after his loss, he had a picture of the baby's profile silhouette tattooed on his forearm. He wanted to feel connected to his baby. What he didn't expect was that it would create such a web of interconnection and compassion.

Since he was a mechanic in a large detailing shop, he came in contact with many people every day. Frequently, both men and women commented on his tattoo and how interesting it was. This gave Joey an opportunity to share the significance of the tattoo. More often than not, the observer had a similar story of either themselves or someone they knew who had endured the pain of miscarriages, stillbirths, and infant deaths.

Joey began to see his baby's life—and his own willingness to share about his baby—as a connector to others and a vehicle for normalizing and discussing loss. The baby's influence spread to something more, creating opportunities for others to connect and heal. When feeling especially overcome by grief, Joey could shift to the Light of this powerful effect rather than just focusing on the pain of his loss.

Remember kintsugi, the Japanese art form of repairing broken pottery pieces with gold lacquer? The result is a stunning piece of art that honors precious scars, that celebrates beauty in the broken places. Kintsugi recognizes the grace of the new form that arises out of brokenness, a spiritual alchemy of sorts. The gold (Spirit) shines amidst the brokenness (grief) leading to a new luminosity. Something more than the sum of its parts arises.

Leonard Cohen, poet and lyricist, popularized the idea that there's a crack in everything but that's how the Light gets in. I would suggest that there's a crack, yes, but that's how the *gold* Light gets in. Spiritual gold.

The next section of the book discusses four Lightshift Divine qualities that help you alchemize your grief, each an experience of Light: Love, Connection, Compassion, and Faith.

LIGHT-SHIFT PRACTICES

1—Grief Graph

In cognitive-behavioral therapy, clients are often advised to chart their moods and keep track of the ups and downs. We can think we know what's happening emotionally in our lives, but until we put it on paper, we often don't realize the trends. It's helpful to see emotional content translated onto a chart, in color or black and white, so that we can make some sense out of what otherwise feels chaotic, by tracking movement over time.

The Practice

Get a large piece of blank or graph paper and create a chart for yourself. On the left-hand side, write the numbers 1 to 10, with 1 at the bottom and 10 at the top. For measurement, 1 is deeply depressed and 10 is feeling great. At the bottom of the page, horizontally, make hash marks 1 cm apart, each designating a consecutive day of the month. At the end of the day, starting on the left, rate your mood for the day by placing a dot at the appropriate height above the hash mark. Add new pages as necessary. Start to notice the trend over time. You might have a LOT of days in the 1 to 3 range over the first few months. Then, you'll notice days getting into the 4–6 range. You might have a 1 day from time to time, but you will see that they gain space between them. You might even start to notice days over a 7 as time goes by.

2—Turn It Over

There are all kinds of prayers in this world: prayers of requests/supplications (for self), prayers of petition or intercession (on behalf of others), prayers of praise, of thanksgiving, of devotion, of consecration. There are formal prayers (Our Father, Hail Mary) and prayers that are simply words from your heart.

There is also a prayer of oblation—a kind of presentation or offering to a Higher Power. With grief, the offering is our own state of suffering. Give your grief over and ask for help. In twelve-step programs, they talk about "turning over" your addiction, your burden, your struggle, to a Higher Power. It's too much to handle on your own. Allow that which is greater than yourself to carry this burden with you, for you.

In her beautiful book, *Help Thanks Wow,* Anne Lamott says that in general, there are only three essential prayers to utter. Help! is one of those prayers, and the time is now.

The Practice

Close your eyes. Picture Light flooding down upon you. Say in your mind, "Source Energy. Please help me with my grief. It feels unbearable at times. Please help me bear it. I cannot do it on my own. Help!" And if that feels like too much to say, simply utter the word, "Help!"

Open your hands to the universe, palms up, acknowledging your surrender. Say, "I turn my grief over to you."

Be still. Be silent. Offer your burden. Know that it has been received. You are not alone.

3—Sacred Place

Guided visualizations are a way of calming the nervous system and taking oneself on a journey of the heart. After spending a few minutes imagining yourself in a place that feels safe and peaceful, a place where your heart is full, your body and mind react as if you had actually been to this place. So go ahead and take yourself on a sentimental journey.

The Practice

Begin by settling yourself in a comfortable place and position. Close your eyes and let yourself breathe deeply for several rounds of breath. Then imagine a location that feels sacred to you, a place that feels treasured, special, holy, hallowed. It can be a place of physical beauty or a place of intimate familiarity. It can be an imaginary setting or a place as familiar and as comfortable as your own bed. You can go to a different setting each time you do this practice or return to a beloved place over and over.

Immerse yourself in the sensory field of this place—how does it smell, what do you see, what do you hear, what can you touch? Is the air warm or cool on your skin? Are you alone or are there other people around? Do you hear birds, dogs barking, wind, water? How is the light—bright, dim? Let yourself bask in the scene and watch what unfolds. How do you feel visiting this special spot?

After a few minutes—or however long feels comfortable—start to return to the present moment in real time. Wiggle your fingers and toes, orienting you to your current location. Breathe deeply. Touch your arms and put your hand on your heart. Let yourself feel restored and filled by your visit.

4—Hold Me Tight

With trauma, there is often a tendency to disassociate, to "leave the body." This is a protective and adaptive measure, but it also limits our ability to process emotion. In treating trauma, practitioners help clients feel contained in and safe within their bodies again. The following practice is one way to achieve this sense of safety along with the comfort of being held.

The Practice

Place your right hand under your left armpit. Then take your left arm and wrap it around to hug your right arm. Breathe. Notice the edges of your own body. Notice that you are contained and held. You also could add a tender rubbing of your own right arm. Then, add a gentle sway of your body, from left to right, left to right. Let yourself sway to the whispered music of emotion within you.

After a few minutes in this hug hold, come out of it by lightly pinching along your arms from shoulder to wrist and wrist to shoulder, gentle pinches to wake up the skin and alert you to the fact that yes, you are here. You are in this moment. You are present.

5—Voo Chanting

Peter Levine is a trauma specialist who recommends this deep breathing technique as a low belly, high vibrational healing chant. This regulates your nervous system and tones the vagus nerve. If you are experiencing overwhelm and despair (which most grievers feel at some point), this breath chant is extremely effective.

The Practice

Bring your hands to your belly and breathe into the belly, and when you exhale, drop your jaw and make a low sound like a foghorn, "Vooooooooooooooooo." Notice the vibration resonating throughout your body. Do this repeatedly for at least three minutes, breathing in while expanding your belly and then breathing out on the low chant, "Voooo." Three minutes of this deep breathing actually changes oxygen levels in the blood and stimulates the parasympathetic nervous system (the rest and digest system of the body).

Notice how your body responds. Now, breathe normally and see if your body registers a sense of more calm.

PART 2:

THE SPIRITUAL HEART
OF COMFORT AND HOPE

*You are not a drop in the ocean. You are the
entire ocean in a drop.*

—*RUMI*

I once posed the following question to my Facebook community, "Transcending Loss" —*What Surprises You about Your Grief*? The most consistent response from over one hundred replies was one of astonishment, astonishment that grief still continues after many years. Until they experienced their own loss, they didn't realize that grief would sneak up on them year after year, even after decades. Grief might change and transform, but it never goes away. Even the most painful parts can return when you least expect it.

Collectively we hold the myth that grief has an end, that closure is possible. We hope that the funeral will bring closure (actually, it's just the beginning of the journey). We hope that prosecuting or suing someone might bring closure (actually, it only stokes anger and blame). We hope that passing the one-year anniversary might bring closure (actually, believing that will make the second year harder).

Loss never ends because love never ends. Loss and love are two sides of the same coin. They are both a part of you. Yet this doesn't mean that your grief will remain unbearable. Grief is always changing, softening, aging. It is a lifelong process of healing and growth.

Fortunately, there are ways to cope, to lessen the pain, to hasten the healing. There are ways to make bad better. There are Light-shift strategies that help bring the vertical dimension of life into focus and harness the support of an illuminated world within and beyond yourself.

Synthesis is what I call the ongoing process of living with loss, the art of folding grief into your life. Grief softens, shifts, transmutes, recedes, and at times doubles back again on itself. I first wrote about Synthesis several decades ago in my book, *Transcending Loss*. Synthesis is the arc of grief over time.

Grief will occasionally slice back into your life in a raw form as "grief bursts," even after many years have passed. Because you carry your loved one with you in your heart, periodically the reality of their physical loss will hit you in the gut. Triggered by a sound, a smell, a song, a holiday, a memory, a calendar date—or nothing at all, the pain will slam you. But even as the burst shocks, the burst also reminds you of love and the tender relationship that enriched and continues to enrich your life.

Part of your journey to Higher Healing is learning to change your relationship to your grief. Instead of seeing it as the enemy, you come at first to see it as the uninvited guest, and then maybe even a friend. Instead of seeing grief as the end of your life, you come to see it as the portal to a vertical dimension to your life. You *accept* loss as it is and see where it's going to take you, or where you want it to take you.

You can't change that your loved one has died, but you can change, bit by bit, how you relate to your grief, how you shift toward the Light of meaning and greater good in your world, and how you choose to live life going forward.

Maybe you've heard the Native American Indian story about the two wolves. A Cherokee elder was teaching his grandson about life. "Everyone has two wolves inside of them and there is a fight between them," he said. "The evil wolf is angry, sad, arrogant, resentful, selfish, and full of self-pity." He continued, "The other wolf, the good wolf, is full of joy, peace, hope, happiness, generosity, compassion, faith, and serenity."

He finished with, "And this same fight between these wolves is going on inside of you and inside of every person."

The grandson thought about this and asked, "Which wolf will win?"

The Cherokee elder replied simply, "The one that you feed."

What you feed grows. What you put your attention on expands. You will always have choices on your journey through life. Do you focus on loss or love, on absences or presence, on tears or smiles, on the horizontal or the vertical, on darkness or Light? On the grief journey, especially in the beginning, it is important to honor the loss and pain. But also, and increasingly over time, opportunities arise to shift your attention to the Light, to the love, joys, smiles, and meaning in your life. There will be some days when you will have more energy and purpose, and other days in which you will barely get off of the couch.

The following four chapters are each focused on the vertical, divine experiences of Love, Connection, Compassion, and Faith. Each is a kind of spiritual glue—the gold glue of kintsugi—that leads to higher healing. Each Light-shift transforms grief into something more than just pain or suffering.

You may find that you lean toward one or more of these four divine experiences early and often in your grief process. Or it may take some time. Be patient; there is no rush.

You may find that one divine aspect is easier for you to embody than the others. That's fine too. Go with what is natural and comfortable for you in the time frame that feels right for you. Also, you may find that these experiences change over time. The way you inhabit love, connection, compassion, or faith may look one way in the first year of your grief but look very different after the fifth year of your grief.

Grief over time becomes a toggling between *being with* the darkness and *lifting* one's gaze to the Light . . . between looking down and looking up . . . between the shadowed horizontal experience of painful grief and the illuminated vertical experience of healing and spiritual awareness.

With each intentional Light-shift, you start to tap into the divine experiences of love, connection, compassion, and faith and find that grief is leading you on a path toward higher consciousness. These vantage points are the places where you develop a new relationship with your grief. Grief morphs from enemy to companion. Intentionally plugging into that which is holy in your life will comfort, carry, and elevate you along your life-long journey of living with loss.

CHAPTER 3
LOVE

Love is the bridge between you and everything.
—RUMI

Imagine that I had a magic wand and I came to you with a deal: "I can wave my wand and make all of your sorrow and pain and grief disappear in an instant. There will be no more tears, no more longing, no more missing your loved one. But there is a catch: as I take away the pain, I will also take away your memory. It will be as if you never met, knew, or loved your dear one. You will have no sense of their presence (or absence) anymore. YOU as you are now will be untouched by their influence, their impact, their love pressed upon you. To you, they will never have existed. No loved one. No grief."

Would you accept this proposition?

Alfred Tennyson wouldn't have. He modeled

accepting grief in the face of love in his famous 1850
poem "In Memoriam: 27":

> *I hold it true, whate'er befall;*
> *I feel it, when I sorrow most.*
> *It's better to have loved and lost*
> *than never to have loved at all.*

Even with the pain of loss, you are buoyed by the
richness, the blessings, the sheer joy of having known
and loved your dear ones. They enriched and magnified
your life; your mutual love shapes the "you" who you
currently are. For most, the love far outweighs the cost
of heartbreak. Love is a package deal but, in the end, it's
worth the price. Don't you think?

ALL YOU NEED IS LOVE

The reason grief is so painful is because love is so deep
and vast. Whether you knew your dear one for sixty
seconds or sixty years, they touched your heart. The
good news is that while a physical body can die, love
does not die. Love is eternal.

And while love is the reason for the grief, love is the
reason for the warmth in your heart as well. Over time,
sharp sorrow softens to a sweet sorrow, and you start to
get a smile before you get a tear.

Love cannot be taken from you. It grows; it expands.
Turning your focus to the love is a profound Light-shift.

Margie told me that she feels closer to her grandfather now, since he had passed. "When Papa was alive, I was so busy with my life that I could only call him about once a month."

"Now," she continued, "I talk to him more often, every day, especially when I look at his photo and feel his presence all around me. I know he is with me, and I love him more than ever."

The body is simply a garment, an earth suit. The essence of the person who died is still very present. You simply have to find a new way to relate to the formless, to demonstrate your love and receive theirs in return.

Whether you believe that their soul has moved on to another realm, reincarnated, rejoined the natural cycle of nature, or reentered the universal life energy, you keep them alive through your memories and stories.

Some of the ways to engage their essence:

- Talk out loud to your loved one
- Blow kisses to their photograph
- Pray for them
- Visualize them during a meditation
- Visit the gravesite and leave a flower or stone
- Give gifts to others in their honor
- Share stories about them
- Recite the Mourner's Kaddish (a Jewish tradition)

The mourner's prayer, the Kaddish, is spoken collectively during a worship service to remind each mourner that they are not alone. It has been said for over two thousand years in the Jewish tradition. Traditionally, the kaddish is said daily for eleven months after the passing of a parent and then annually, on each anniversary of their death.

When you nurture your love relationship with your dear one, you are less envious of others who have their loved ones still on the planet. It's not unusual to find it difficult to watch others in happy circumstances when you're grieving. It can be hard, for example, if you're a widow watching other couples, or if you're a bereaved parent watching other families with children.

However, when you shift your focus to the Light of the love that you shared and still have, the love that is still a part of you, you can start to make a shift.

I once had the fun experience of wearing a hoop skirt and ball gown on stage while singing a gorgeous song from *The King and I* to a packed audience. The Rodgers and Hammerstein classic, "Hello Young Lovers," is sung by Anna, a widow who is happy to see other young lovers living their lives. She doesn't begrudge them for their happiness, realizing that she too has known such a sweet love. She is happy for others to know the joy that she has known.

For each of us, the trick is to remember the love you had and still have (imprinted within you) so that you focus on the love that still lives in your heart, rather than focusing on what you've lost.

One way to do this is through self-talk, again and again. Even as you are sad, put your hand over your heart and say, "I know this is hard but don't forget that what you had was a great love, a great joy, and it will always be a part of you, now and always." Another way is to look at photographs of good times (perhaps holidays and vacations), and say to yourself, "Those were amazing times. You were so lucky to have that experience. It will always be woven within you."

Your heart may be broken, but when you put the pieces back together with the gold of spiritual awareness, you will see that your heart can beat even more vibrantly. You're able to focus more on love and not simply loss. Love is the reason we are here on this planet. It is stronger than death and needs to be shared. Can you let your loved one shine through you as an expression of love? Can you hold it, expand it, and share that love with others still here?

LOVE FOR THE LIVING

On a sunny afternoon in New Hampshire, right in the middle of a park, I gathered with a handful of people for a granite bench dedication. We were there to honor the life of a young girl who had died. The bench was being dedicated in her memory.

However, what struck me about this brief ceremony

was that the minister presiding took the opportunity to honor the child's two surviving brothers. The minister talked about Johanna who had died from cancer. But even as he honored Johanna's memory, he implored us to turn our attention to the living. Then, he asked the brothers to come up, place a rose on the bench, and then to sit on the bench. I still remember his final words: "Do not forget those who have departed this earth. But for heaven's sake, don't forget those who are still here."

His message was clear to all of us: staying connected to the deceased does not mean a pass on staying connected to those still living. We need each other and we need community. Finding ways to share and engage with larger groups of people, people with similar interests and passions, whether in person or online, helps us to feel more integrated and hopeful.

However, if you're not feeling ready to connect with others just yet, that's fine. If you are feeling more introverted, it's okay to dose your time with others. Take the time you need to stay in your own internal process of noticing and experiencing your grief (in addition to savoring the love that you hold in your heart). Again, you must tend to the grief even as you tend to the love. Be patient with the process and give yourself time for shifts to occur.

Remember that you may take one step forward and then two steps backward, and that's part of the journey. Perhaps the idea of your heart expanding is simply a seed at the moment. So, plant the seed and wait . . . wait . . . watch it bloom in its time.

KAHLIL GIBRAN, "THE PROPHET"

You would know the secret of death.

But how shall you find it unless you seek it in the heart of life?

The owl whose night-bound eyes are blind unto the day cannot unveil the mystery of Light.

If you would indeed behold the spirit of death, open your heart wide unto the body of life.

For life and death are one, even as the river and the sea are one.

LOVE AS FORGIVENESS

Every now and then, I'll hear an incredible story of forgiveness that demonstrates an almost other-worldly tale of agape love. Before I tell you the story of Elaine Prevallet, as told in her book *Toward a Spirituality for Global Justice*, I want to define a few terms, beginning with the word *forgiveness*. Forgiveness is not about condoning a terrible or even reprehensible act. Forgiveness is a personal process that liberates the forgiver from the corrosive weight of resentment and anger.

The term *agape* refers to a higher love, an unconditional love, one that transcends the needs of the ego and requires no thanks or praise as payment. It is love for love's sake, regardless of circumstances. From the Greco-Christian tradition, the concept of agape describes the "highest love," as experienced with deep compassion, sacrificial love, and altruism. Agape love is thought to be reflected in Jesus's love for the world, or in the lives of those who serve selflessly, such as Mother Teresa. It is distinguished from other types of love, such as brotherly love (philia), erotic love (eros), or self-love (philautia).

Elaine was a victim of apartheid in South Africa. Both her husband and only son were killed by white men right in front of her. When her husband died, he echoed the words of Jesus on the cross, saying, "Father, forgive them."

She faced the perpetrators of these crimes during the "Truth and Reconciliation Commission," a court-like restorative justice body assembled so that those accused of the crimes had to face their victims and the families of victims.

It was in such a courtroom that Elaine faced the security officer who had confessed to murdering her husband and son. Echoing her husband's example of an open heart, she told the courtroom that she wanted only three things: (1) to see where her husband's body had been buried, and (2) for the perpetrator to know that she forgave him.

Number 3 was a more complicated request. She said that she had a lot of love in her heart to give to a son, but she no longer had a son. So she requested that he visit with her every week, like a son, to talk with her and share their days.

Upon hearing this, the man collapsed in the courtroom with tears. She went up to him for a hug and suddenly, a chorus of "Amazing Grace" filled the room, beginning with one voice and spreading to every voice in the room. What they all witnessed was indeed amazing grace.

Elaine was able to rise to this level of agape love because she asked for God's help and invited her husband's spirit, already an exemplar of forgiveness, to be present with her. For any of us, aspiring to agape love is usually a process in which we need to relax our story of self and let Spirit flow through us. Often, asking for divine assistance is helpful.

Another example of awe-inspiring open-hearted forgiveness is that of Immaculee Ilbagiza. She survived the Rwanda Genocide in 1994 by hiding with seven other women in a tiny bathroom (only three feet by four feet) for ninety-one days. During that time, most of her family was murdered (her mother, her father, and two brothers). In her book *Left to Tell,* she describes how her Catholic faith guided her through her unspeakable trauma and helped her find forgiveness and compassion toward the killers.

In her second book, *Led by Faith,* she describes how her faith in God helped her find peace again. Now, she speaks all over the world and leads retreats and pilgrimages. She has a mission of encouraging and inspiring people all over the world to survive and find peace. She shares that forgiveness is a pathway to inner peace.

Something beyond the self needs to intervene to

heal such a deep wound and facilitate a turn toward the Light. Basically, you have to get your ego out of the way for such a profound healing to take place. Miranda Macpherson is a spiritual teacher who describes a process of what she calls "ego relaxation" in order to invite space for forgiveness.

In her book, *The Way of Grace*, she describes how when you regard everything as a divine invitation, you can relax the ego by opening, softening, allowing. This repetitive process of opening, softening, and allowing leads to an experience of presence, or grace, in which you can melt. When you connect with this energy—when you know that you are not the "doer"—forgiveness becomes natural.

Spirit and love are the ingredients to create such a thorough restoration. Spirit and love are what will help you turn toward your higher healing.

Love is Spiritual Light in the cracks of your grief.

LIGHT-SHIFT PRACTICES

1—Wisdom Council

Sometimes we cannot summon wisdom on our own, but we can imagine wisdom coming from a beloved or revered person.

The Practice
Close your eyes and visualize a calm place. It could be a garden, down by a river, on the beach, in a church. Now, shift to the Light of someone to whom you feel a strong connection. For example, your grandmother or grandfather, the Buddha, Jesus, the Virgin Mary, a deceased relative, your mother or father, the Dalai Lama, a favorite minister, priest, or rabbi, a favorite teacher or mentor, Gandhi, Mother Teresa, Martin Luther King Jr. Visualize bringing one or more people into the scene and either walk or sit beside them.

Feel their energy next to you. Imagine what they might say to you, if anything. Notice whether you have much to say or very little to say. Simply let yourself relax into their presence. Notice their agape smile, their warm gaze, their loving nature. Stay there as long as it feels comfortable.

Next, bring yourself back into your room in real time. Notice how you feel after your "visit."

2–Treasure Chest of Memories
Photographs tell a story. They remind you of a time, a place, a moment frozen in time. I have always loved photographs, both as an art form and as a visual journal of life. While photographs can initially cause a painful feeling, a sense of heightened absence, photographs can also serve as a catalyst for happy memories, a cause for celebration of the good in your life, and a vehicle for remembering love.

The Practice

Search your own photo albums. Photographs of your own life, of past vacations, of times with your loved one are a double-edged sword. They might cause a sharp sadness as the absence of this person is brought to your attention. But if you stay with that feeling, see if it can soften to a different sensation.

Look at this person, the Light in their eyes and their participation in this moment. Remember what it felt like to be living the moment captured by the photograph. Close your eyes and see if you can savor the feeling, locating the emotion in your body. See if gratitude can overlay any sorrow as you realize how lucky you were to have such a moment. Ahhhhhhhh.

3—Thank You, Dear One

Even though you are feeling a wide range of painful feelings on your grief journey, you want to encourage your mind to remember and focus both on the love that you had (and continue to have) for your dear one, and on the love that they had for you.

Love is a two-way street—their love affected your soul and your love affected theirs. Their love is imprinted upon your heart. The next time you feel a tinge of sorrow, or simply have a memory that makes you smile, focus on and expand the feeling of love.

Know that today still has their presence contained within it. You could say that you live with an absence/presence, which is far better than living with an absence/absence.

Fate brought you together for some reason. And now, your dear ones are with you always in your heart and soul. You cannot be without them, actually. So be aware of love, intentionally and gratefully, with the following practice.

The Practice
Put your hand over your heart. Close your eyes, breathe, and say out loud,

"Thank you, thank you, _____ (name of loved one), my dear one. Thank you for your love which is imprinted upon me and within me. Thank you for the opportunity to be formed and molded by your love. And thank you for giving me the opportunity to love you, which I will do for all the rest of my days."

Breathe in the feeling of their love toward you. Breathe out the feeling of your love toward them. Again, breathe in the feeling of their love for you. Breathe out the feeling of your love for them. Open your eyes. Let love fill you, overflowing from your heart space.

4—Ho'oponopono

This ancient Hawaiian practice is about reconciliation and forgiveness. The direct translation into English means "correction." You can think of it as a kind of karmic cleansing, a purification. Use it to clear your mind so that you can do good things in the world and not get tripped up with anger and resentment.

The following sentences tap into the human experiences of repentance, forgiveness, love, and gratitude.

The Practice
Repeat these sentences ten times, out loud:

- I'm sorry.
- Forgive me.
- I love you.
- Thank you.

In broadcasting this energy to the Universe, it is said that you will experience compassion and a relaxed mind. You will clear negative blocks, neutralize traumatic cell memory, and release resentments. Now you are free to dwell in the Spiritual experience of pure love.

5—Love Sponge
Neuroscience has shown that repetition is essential for creating new neural pathways. But another technique makes the process go faster: amplification. Amplification is when you use your mind to really heighten the recall of an experience, using details to deepen the intensity.

This tool uses imagination and a breath mantra to enhance and amplify your experience of love.

The Practice
Take in the Love: Imagine the love that you know and see if you can **feel** it in your body. As you continue to

breathe naturally, breathe in "Love." What does it feel like to love someone and be loved? What does it feel like to have known your loved one? As you breathe out naturally, breathe out "Pain." Breathe in LOVE. Breathe out "suffering." Breathe in LOVE—and imagine absorbing it into your cells, as if you are a dry and thirsty sponge. Breathe out pain and suffering, giving it space and distance from you. Breathe in the Light of LOVE. Feel it. Breathe out the darkness of grief. Let it go.

CHAPTER 4

CONNECTION

*Anything you lose comes round in
another form.*

—RUMI

I was in junior high when I learned that a mushroom was more than an oddity in the woods, a fairy umbrella or an ingredient in a creamy soup. To my fascination, I discovered that a mushroom is the visible expression of a vast underground root network. This network is so vast, in fact, that it spreads throughout the forest floor carrying nutrients for miles and miles. Years later, I would watch the documentary *Fantastic Fungi* and be reminded of how the mushroom's underground network connects our landscape and has done so for hundreds of millions of years.

Just as when you're in a motorboat cruising through

ocean waters above a vast, integrated world teeming with life. So too, whenever you walk in the woods, you're walking over a whole world of life—animal homes, insect colonies, tree roots and, yes, a wide-reaching mushroom net. Nature abounds, all of its visible aspects united by unseen connections.

CONNECTING TO NATURE

I once heard a speaker talking about the benefits of "forest bathing." Forest bathing is a phenomenon that originated in Japan (called shinrin-yoku) that takes the art of spending time outdoors to a new level. Walking in nature, especially amongst trees, and intentionally soaking in the environment through all of our senses calms a person's nervous system.

Forest bathing is not your average walk in the woods. It's a therapeutic immersion practice done slowly, silently, and without technology. The healing comes in part from a mindful intention to really soak in the forest environment. The instruction is multisensory: Notice your feet on the ground. Listen to the sounds of the forest. Look at the colors around you. Look for things you can see but not hear. Look down. Look up. Inhale deeply. Touch tree bark and flower petals. Feel the air on your skin. Notice your breathing.

Dr. Qing Li, the author of *Forest Bathing: How Trees Can Help You Find Health and Happiness*, relates how therapeutic phytoncides produced by trees enhance our white blood cell count, thereby boosting our immune systems. Forest bathing is also linked to improved sleep, better health, and stress reduction.

Actually, ecosystems of all types have a powerful effect on the body, mind, and spirit: gardens, fields and meadows, oceans, lakes. We feel at home with nature because we are, in fact, a part of nature.

In so many ways, we *crave* nature. We long for it. We yearn for green space (trees, plants, forests), blue space (lakes, oceans, rivers), and wide-open vistas (mountains, sunsets, stars). Why? Because it connects us to that which is beyond ourselves, to something bigger, something more.

I have often spoken with people who say that they don't believe in "God," but they feel completely at peace and calm and connected when they float on a lake or sit by the ocean or walk a trail in the forest. Resistance floats away as they feel part of a greater whole, as they shift their attention and connect to a vertical dimension in life. In truth, connecting with nature *is* a spiritual experience. You're connecting to the infinite ground of grace.

The plants and trees and animals and insects are all part of a delicate ecosystem of which we are a part and in which we all depend on each other. Trees, reaching for the sun, are literal reminders of the vertical dimension—deep roots that drink in nourishment from the earth, and high branches, stretching toward the Light.

I once listened to a minister ask his congregation, "Do you know where most people find Spirit, the Eternal, the ground of our Being?" We shook our heads. "Is it in the grand cathedrals of Europe? The small churches in rural New England? The mosques or temples or ashrams around the world?"

"No," he continued. "Most people find that they connect to a Higher Power when they are out in nature." Yes. We feel the aliveness, the energy, the life force of something vast and powerful when we connect with the natural world. Nature is quintessentially vertical.

When I worked with George, a seventy-two-year-old man who was grieving the loss of his cat, his best friend of twenty-one years, he walked in the woods every day for six months in order to heal. He told me, "I have lost pets before, and been completely devastated. But back then I didn't hike, you know? I never knew how I would survive the loss of Ginger but now I get it— it's the woods, the being in nature that helps me feel connected to her and to all things—it's helping me heal in a way that I didn't expect."

He also told me that his favorite part of each hike is when he finds a tree to lean on. "I know it sounds crazy, but when my back leans up against a tree, right when I feel the bark, I just start to feel better."

Nature not only embraces us as part of a larger whole but connects us to the cycles of life and death. Nature reminds us that there is a greater energy that moves beyond space and time. Turning toward the natural world is a Light-shift that brings Spirit into full view; it is a portal to our everlasting connection to our loved ones.

NATURE AS THE CONDUIT

I sat shoulder to shoulder with a group of musicians. For the second time in a year, we were singing at a funeral for a loved one connected to our musical family. First, someone old and now, someone young—death felt present amongst us.

We sang a beautiful arrangement of the following Mary Frye poem, "Do Not Stand at My Grave and Weep":

> *Do not stand at my grave and weep*
> *I am not there; I do not sleep.*
> *I am a thousand winds that blow,*
> *I am the diamond glints on snow,*
> *I am the sun on ripened grain,*
> *I am the gentle autumn rain.*
> *When you awaken in the morning's hush*
> *I am the swift uplifting rush*
> *Of quiet birds in circled flight.*
> *I am the soft stars that shine at night.*
> *Do not stand at my grave and cry,*
> *I am not there; I did not die.*

I couldn't get through the song without tears streaming down my cheeks, making it hard to read the music. The idea of a soul being expressed through nature, the idea that no one really "dies," the feeling of ongoing connection to the awesome beauty of this glorious, interconnected world opened my heart and moved me to tears.

Shamans and indigenous peoples around the world have revered nature as the Great Spirit, the Great Mystery. Pagan and Wiccan rituals honor the rhythms of the earth, from solstices to seasons. And in the Bible, in Genesis, it says, "Then God said, 'Let the earth sprout vegetation, plants yielding seed, and fruit trees on the earth bearing fruit after their kind with seed in them', and it was so. The earth brought forth vegetation, plants yielding seed after their kind, and trees bearing fruit with seed in them, after their kind; and God saw that it was good."

Nature is creation, mystery, beauty and, potentially, a conveyor from the beyond. Often, I have heard psychics share things like, "The great eagle you saw circling over your house last week was your husband communicating with you." Cardinals, butterflies, dragonflies, hummingbirds, owls—when these and other animals behave in unusual ways around you, or seem to come out of nowhere, they seem to have a message in communicating that a loved one's spirit is nearby.

CONNECTING TO YOUR LOVED ONE

For many decades, the prevailing "wisdom" of grief theory was a focus on closure, acceptance, and moving on. There was no emphasis on maintaining ties with the deceased. Now, happily, we understand the vital role of nurturing continuing bonds with your loved one. Just because a person's body has died does not mean that the relationship is over.

Quite the contrary. While a physical relationship has ended, an emotional and spiritual relationship continues.

Here are healthy ways that people honor their ongoing connection to their loved one:

- talk out loud to your loved one
- talk to others about your loved one, keeping their memory alive
- cook dishes that your loved one cooked or loved to eat
- visit the grave site and put flowers or stones there
- look at photographs prominently displayed in your home
- make a quilt or pillow with their clothes
- ask your friends for stories about your loved one
- get a tattoo that makes you feel connected to your loved one

Another way to stay connected to your loved one is to do things that they would do: bake their famous cookie recipe, go to an event that they would have enjoyed (in their honor), take a trip that they had wanted to take.

In the 2010 movie, *The Way*, Martin Sheen plays the

role of a father who completes the pilgrimage to Spain's Santiago de Compostela after his estranged son dies while making the same journey. The son is played by the actor Emilio Estevez (who, interestingly, is Martin Sheen's son in real life). As the movie unfolds, the father takes his son's ashes and spreads them along the road of the Camino. He completes the journey that his son wasn't able to make and, in the process, comes to understand both himself and his son in a new way. In this instance, the father felt closer to his son in death than he had in life. It's never too late to develop a relationship.

BEYOND THIS WORLD

I love to visit Star Island, a small rock of an island seven miles off the coast of New Hampshire and Maine. I have been traveling there every summer for twenty years. They say it's a "thin place," a place where the veil between this world and the next is delicate and permeable, an atmosphere for divine connection. The Celtic saints referred to thin places, mostly in Ireland and Scotland, in which there were spiritual portals— places of no barriers between heaven and earth. Other geographic pilgrimage destinations are considered thin places with miraculous properties: Iona, Lourdes, Medjugorje, Bodh Gaya, Guadeloupe, and Jerusalem, to name a few.

For me, when I'm on Star, I have a mystical feeling that ghosts are about, as if I can almost see and hear the fishermen village's eighteenth-century inhabitants who prayed in the same chapel that now stands on the highest point of the island.

Of course, no one can really prove the experience of ghosts, spirits, the beyond, eternity. What actually happens after death is truly a mystery. Still, we hear consistent stories from people who have had NDEs (near death experiences) as well as consistent stories from psychic mediums who communicate with the dearly departed. And we hear some interesting stories from people who have had past life regressions as well.

While Christians and Muslims believe in heaven, Buddhists and Hindus believe in reincarnation. Albert Einstein confirmed that energy cannot be either created or destroyed (the First Law of Thermodynamics)—that energy simply changes from one form to another but does not disappear. But where does that energy go?

Clearly, there is much uncertainty and much that occurs beyond what we can see or understand. I once spoke with a rabbi who told me that his religion prefers the term "afterlife." He said, with something of a twinkle in his eye, "There is certainly an *after* even if we don't know exactly what it is. But I bet it's pretty wonderful. Spectacular even."

I know for myself that I embrace Mystery. And when I'm at Star Island connecting with land, sky, and sea, I do feel a shift to the Light, "Something More" in a profound way. But the truth is that you don't need to be in a thin place to communicate with the other side of the veil. All you need is a willingness, an open heart, and an open mind.

Josephine looked quite troubled as she sat across from me in my office. She put her head down, sheepishly, and looked at her hands in her lap. She said, "I don't know how to say this and I'm pretty sure that you'll think that I'm crazy ... but ... several times a day this smell comes out of nowhere, and it's just on my right shoulder ... it's *really strong,* and it makes me think of her."

Josephine was not the sort of person who believed in spirits, and yet she was having a common experience in connecting with a deceased loved one.

I normalized and honored her experience that it was likely a message from Jill, her twin sister who had died two months previously. For Josephine, her relationship with her twin had been powerful, intense, and sustaining. I told her that signs and a feeling of presence were not unusual. To experience something like this was a gift.

She looked at me incredulously. "But what makes you think it's real ... how do you know?"

I told her that I can't know for sure other than that it feels true in my bones. And, I have heard stories for thirty years of people who have had signs and who have communicated with loved ones through psychic mediums and channelers.

One could argue that a griever who attends a psychic session is simply desperate for some message from the beyond and will believe virtually anything. But I have heard reports of specific details, of unknowable knowings, and highly individualized messages that have made me a believer.

I have also studied Eastern traditions that describe past lives, reincarnation, the bardo state (when consciousness is between this life and the next), and karmic debts over lifetimes. So, I hold the general assumption that what we see and experience with our five senses is simply not the whole picture. There is more to our existence than what can be perceived or explained.

I myself have received signs from dear ones in the form of songs on the radio, white feathers, dreams, and pennies from heaven. The most common forms of signs that I have heard of from others include dream visitations, warmth on the skin or a cool blast on the skin, distinct smells, songs on the radio, unusual electric activity (lights on and off, computers on and off), feathers, and animal sightings (usually birds or butterflies).

I have even had the distinct honor, on quite a few occasions, to feel the presence of spirits in my office, right in the room with me and my client even as we discuss them. It always feels warm, loving, and supportive. At this point in my career, I'm pretty open to the fact that anything is possible, even if it doesn't seem logical.

I especially appreciate the beautiful Latin American celebration on November 1–2 known as the Day of the

Dead (Día de los Muertos), in which families gather in homes, cemeteries, and community spaces to honor their departed loved ones. The multiday ritual focuses on celebrating and connecting, obviously cherishing the ongoing relationship with the deceased. It is said that the souls of the dead come back to visit their loved ones during this time, and there is a palpable sense that the living and the dead are having a festive reunion.

Families take decorations, photographs, and feasts to the cemetery—special food dishes and beverages—as gifts, or offerings, for their ancestors. Some people even spend all night in the cemetery amidst a carnival-like atmosphere. For two days, there are processions, elaborate costumes, special breads and candies (sugar skulls), music, and marigolds in the streets—all a celebration of the connection to those who have passed.

THROUGH THE YEARS

Debbie's adult son was brutally murdered by a disgruntled employee. Debbie described feeling hopeless and depressed for over four years. However, she began to experience a Light-shift when she decided to construct a labyrinth in her large backyard. A labyrinth, unlike a maze, has one path in—leading to a center—and the same path out.

Debbie commissioned a local boy scout troop to help her create the labyrinth, using large river stones to create the pathway. The entire point of the labyrinth was to honor Charles, her son. She used the classic Chartres cathedral design and created a weatherproof altar in the center, along with a small wooden seat. Charles was a beloved figure in their small town, so she opened the space to friends and family who might want to walk it when they needed moments of quiet contemplation or when they were missing Charles.

I spoke to Debbie fifteen years after Charles's death. She told me, "I still get so much peace when I walk the labyrinth. And I feel close to Charles, as if he's there with me." She continued, "Often when I sit in the center, I feel his presence. It's either a feeling, or a dragonfly, or some little sign that he's with me."

She said that it was especially moving to see that others had come and left a stone or flower in the center, in honor of Charles. Every year she adds a little something on the path—a fairy or angel figurine, a wind-chime, a bird bath or hummingbird feeder. "Now it's sort of a magical and whimsical place for the whole community, a place for rest and rejuvenation. When I sit here and remember Charles, I don't feel as much pain. I just feel the love."

CONNECTION TO YOUR HIGHER SELF

Each of us is made up of many internal parts. There is the part of you that is crushed and broken and singed by the fires of grief. And there is a part of you, perhaps, that is afraid or angry or remorseful. But there is also a part of you that is more than an ego, more than a human being, even. There is a part of you that is a divine Light. an essence connected to the greater Spirit.

And that part of you knows that you haven't been left. That part is wise and intuitive, strong and centered. That part of you, even if you're not in touch with it, is unshakeable and unchanging. It is your true core, your essence, the vertical aspect of you.

To get in touch with your Higher self, close your eyes. Picture yourself in a stream of white Light that is cascading down onto you and into you through the top of your head. Now imagine stepping away from yourself yet watching your "light infused" self. See yourself radiating and shimmering with Light. This is one way to imagine and access your higher self.

Chelsea Hanson, author of *The Sudden Loss Survival Guide,* found that she had to access her higher self in order to heal. Chelsea was twenty-eight when her mother died.

She says, "When my mother died many years ago, I could relate to being motherless. I believed that my mom was permanently gone and I was motherless.

No wonder I was so sad. This belief brought me tremendous pain."

She continued, "But that was my experience *then*. There are no rights or wrongs in grief, only what's happening in the current moment. Meanings change. Words that upset you now may not another time. You grow, evolve, and adapt as you integrate loss into your life. I have compassion for my younger self, who was doing the best she could."

Over time, Chelsea identified less with her ego self and more with her Higher self.

"As time passed and I learned more about healing," she said, "I came to realize that Mom was not gone. She had changed forms—moving from the physical realm to the spiritual realm. I realized I could hold onto her love, spirit, essence. . . . She was still with me, but in a new, albeit different form. Not physically but spiritually in my heart, mind, and soul. Our relationship continued."

She continued, "This new belief brought solace rather than suffering. Our love grows and expands. Her spirit is in how I raise my son, how I live my life, and how I value the preciousness of each day. She is my mother. She will always be my mother. And I will always be her daughter. I am not motherless. I continue to love her in the present moment. Love transcends even death. Our relationship is based on the continuing bonds of deep love."

Chelsea still misses her mom, of course. And surely would prefer for her mother to be here on planet Earth. But Chelsea knows that she shifts toward the Light as she identifies more and more with her own Higher Self, her Divine self. And there, she can more easily connect with her mother's spirit.

Connection is Spiritual Light in the cracks of your grief.

LIGHT-SHIFT PRACTICES

1—Life and Breath

Your breath connects you to Spirit. In Hebrew, the word for spirit, *Ruah,* means breath. The Latin root word of spirit, *spir,* also means breath. Deep breathing activates the body's relaxation response. It calms the central nervous system, both grounding and relaxing your mind, opening you to Something More. A breathing exercise is a perfect way to invite Spirit into your life.

With breath, you're connected to all that is. You are one with the plants, with the earth, with the air. This practice helps you connect to a unity greater than yourself.

The Practice

As you stand, lift your body upward by imagining a string at the top of your head pulling you up. Squeeze your shoulder blades slightly together so that your heart center is open and lifted.

Now try what Wiccan priestess and author Phyllis Curott calls "green breathing"—increasing your sense of reverence and unity with the plants around you.

Breathe in—imagine breathing in the oxygen ($O2$) from the green plants, the breath of life for us.

Breathe out—imagine sending carbon dioxide ($CO2$) out to the green plants, the breath of life for them.

Breathe in $O2$, the gift of life from them. Breathe out $CO2$, the gift of life for them.

Continue breathing this way, sharing your CO_2 with the very plants in your area. Intentionally be part of the continuous circle of life, circle of breath, the beautiful complete design of nature, of which you are integral.

The divine awareness of miracle, awareness of unity, is only a breath away.

2—Memory Book

Whenever I talk to someone who is going to a funeral, I suggest that they share with the family any memories of the loved one who died. Grievers love to gather stories of their loved one.

Let's say that you're a widow. You might love to hear stories about your husband's childhood, a time when you didn't know your husband. Or perhaps you would love to hear stories from his colleagues, a work world you perhaps weren't part of during day-to-day interactions.

There is a famous Buddhist story of the blind men and the elephant that illustrates the power of perspective. Each blind man touched a part of the elephant claiming to know what the animal looked like. One said, "This animal is long and thin" (touching the tail); another said, "No it's broad and wide" (touching the ear); while the third blind man said, "This animal is absolutely huge, vast, and rough" (touching the side of the beast).

This practice invites you to gather stories about your loved one from all the different parts of his or her life.

The Practice
Reach out to friends, family members, and colleagues
of your loved one and ask them if they would be willing
to write down memories and stories and send them to
you. You could also ask for photographs. Then, compile
a three-ring binder/notebook in which you include all
of these different stories from different parts of his or
her life.

When you have it all together, you can look through it
at different points in time to feel connected to your loved
one and to know that his/her life touched many people.

3—Ghostwriting

This is a kind of channeling technique that many use to
feel a communication with their dearly departed. Try
this with an open mind. Try it more than once. Just be
open and curious and see what happens.

The Practice
When you have some time to drop into a contemplative
space, try this practice. You may want to light a candle
and have a tissue nearby. Don't rush this process.

With your dominant hand (your writing hand),
write a letter TO your loved one. Tell them how you are
doing, what life is like without them. You could even
ask a question.

With your other, nondominant hand, write a reply
letter FROM your loved one to you. See what comes
through. Using your nondominant hand is designed to

cause the critical, judging brain to be distracted. Again, try not to think too hard about this. Just let something come through you and see what happens.

Some people, for whom this is effective, will use this form of automatic writing on a regular basis to feel connected to their loved one. Automatic writing, or psychography, is known to produce words without consciously writing. You don't need to be a psychic to get the benefits from this technique. All you need is willingness and an open mind.

4—At the Altar

In many traditions, from Asia to Latin America, it is quite customary to have an altar or shrine, a special corner or shelf in the house devoted to honoring loved ones who have passed away. It could be a collection of photos of one's ancestral family tree or it could be a simple candle or bowl full of symbolic trinkets.

Each altar is unique, individualized, and private. It's an intentional place for honoring the memory of someone important to you.

The Practice

Create your own altar. Choose the corner of a room and use a shelf or tray or cabinet to create some magic and mystery in honoring your loved one. Include a photograph if that feels useful. Add symbols of personal meaning: a holy book; natural objects (like shells, stones, or feathers); a candle. Add mala beads or prayer beads or anything that feels reverent and sacred to you.

Now spend some time at your altar. You may bow or namaste to your altar, light a candle, blow a kiss, say a prayer. Use the altar as a way to remember and communicate with your loved one. Say, "My dear one, I send you blessings for happiness. May you be free and at ease wherever you may be. I send love and Light to you."

Let the altar inspire you to continue your loved one's legacy. Use it to check in and evaluate, "What would my dear one think of how I'm grieving?" Or put something on the altar in order to be altered. For example, write your worries or concerns or challenges on a piece of paper and drop it into an offering bowl or dish on your altar. Let the energy of your dear ones assist you just as your energy is assisting them.

5—Signs from Beyond

Lots of people want signs and yet don't feel that they are receiving a sign. The way to ask for a sign, if you wish to receive one, is to take a few moments to drop into a meditative state. Take 5–10 minutes for silence and do the following practice. Take your logical mind out of the equation and allow yourself to open to something more.

The Practice

Sit or lie down in a comfortable position. Read the

following poem from Rumi, the great Sufi poet, mystic, and spiritual teacher of the thirteenth century.

Rumi says:

> *Your body is away from me*
> *but there is a window open*
> *from my heart to yours,*
> *From this window, like the moon*
> *I keep sending news secretly.*

Then, close your eyes and send your news secretly. Summon a picture in your mind's eye of your loved one. Say something along the lines of, "I love you. I am sending you wishes for your peace, your freedom, your joy . . . and I am ready and receptive to receiving any form of communication from you. Please, if you can, let me hear from you. Thank you. I love you."

Here are the key elements of this offering: begin and end your request with an "I love you." Wish them well. State clearly your readiness and receptivity. Know that if they can, they will. And always send your message with a "thank you."

Then, keep your eyes alert for smells, songs, flickering lights, pennies, birds, eagles, feathers, butterflies, hummingbirds, wild animals, cards or letters, invitations, words, dreams. If your loved one can, and you are open, they will send you a sign. Now, surrender the request.

CHAPTER 5
COMPASSION

Don't you know yet? It is your Light
that lights the worlds.

—RUMI

I sat in a circle with fifteen other people, all of whom had experienced their loved one's death by suicide. While I had been invited as a grief expert to share principles about grieving and healing, I had no quick fix to share with them. For each, healing would gather momentum slowly along the unpredictable path of grief. In that moment together, one of the most powerful balms I could offer was to listen and to validate. Every person in the circle knew what it was like to love someone who was in so much pain that they felt they had to exit the planet.

Around the circle, one by one, each person shared their story. And as we listened, there was tenderness.

There was understanding. There was compassion. There was connection. While each loss was unique—a child, a sister, a father, a friend—still every person in the circle seemed to understand the pain of the other.

Everyone, myself included, was in tears when a newly bereaved mother sorrowfully described how she had found her sixteen-year-old son, hanging in the bathroom by his own belt. She was crushed beyond measure.

She said, "I don't even know how to get through the day but mostly I want to know why some of you are still here so many years later after your loss? Is this never going to get any better?"

In response, I shared a bit about how grief doesn't end but it evolves, shifts, and changes. Then Ralph, a bereaved husband of eleven years, gently added, "I come here still, after all these years, because I want to help you. I want to help anyone new to this club that no one wants to join. I want you to know that you're not alone."

At his words, the room was silent for quite a while. This was his gift and also his own healing. It was his Light-shift. In connecting to the pain of another, he came to honor his own pain in the expansiveness of a larger whole. We save ourselves by saving others. This is the power of compassion.

Compassion is the ability to understand and sympathize with the painful feelings of others. It is an essential spiritual practice honored in all religious traditions. We see it embodied by the compassion of Jesus and the Virgin Mary (in the Christian tradition), the compassion of Kwanyin (in the Buddhist tradition), and the compassion of Muhammed (in the Islam tradition), to name just a few.

Compassion is, in essence, a spiritual act. It pulls us into the brilliance of verticality, extending from the depths of our innermost being to heights of connection to that which is greater than ourselves.

COMPASSION FOR OTHER GRIEVERS

I have always loved grief groups. That may sound strange, but truly they are magical. I used to facilitate grief groups in the 1990s in New York City for gay men whose partners and friends had died of AIDS. During those years, I was frequently a guest speaker for groups of bereaved parents and of motherless daughters. I was always amazed by the depth of emotion, the triumphant power of love, and the deep well of compassion that existed among the group members.

It's almost as if an otherworldly energy hangs in the air as the discussion deepens around life and death, the living and the deceased. It is healing to be around people who understand your loss, who get your pain, who have an appreciation for your journey.

While the grieving process itself hasn't changed over time, the ways in which grievers connect with each other has changed. In the 1990s, something new came along to help grievers bond with each other: the internet and social media. The modern world has smartphones, tablets, and laptops that keep us instantly connected to others.

As a result, grievers are able to find each other online, to share stories and offer each other support. Websites, Facebook groups, online courses, YouTube lectures, Instagram—all of these offer support, information, education, and community. It turns out that we are a small world after all, and we can offer compassion to each other with the click of a button.

Jorge and Mitch adopted a daughter from China—an incredible dream come true for them. They adored being dads and were never so happy as when they were with Selina. She was truly their pride and joy.

When Selina was twenty-two years old, she chose to live with an older man of whom neither Mitch nor Jorge approved. However, they wanted Selina to be happy and they tried to be supportive.

That is, until they heard that Dash was physically abusive to Selina. They urged her to end the relationship, but she kept defending Dash's emotional outbreaks. Sadly, one day it was too late. In a burst of anger, Dash picked up a gun and shot Selina. She was killed instantly.

Mitch and Jorge were both devastated, obviously. And yet, they grieved differently—as is often the case. Mitch spent lots of time quietly working in a memorial garden that he planted to honor Selina. He preferred working with his hands, crafting trellises and walkways to add to the garden. For him, connecting to the earth, to plants, and to creativity was where he found solace.

Jorge, on the other hand, needed words to help with his grief expression. He was inconsolable until he found an organization called "Parents of Murdered Children." There he was able to connect with people who understood his pain. He connected with other grievers who had endured unimaginable tragedies—young children murdered by strangers, older children murdered by lovers, and on and on.

Over time, as Jorge shifted to the Light of human connection, he took it upon himself to welcome new members into the Facebook group. He told me that reaching out to these broken people was like a ministry to him, that his heart felt a boundless ocean of compassion for these parents (of which he was one). By helping them, he helped heal his own broken heart.

COMPASSION FOR ALL

Compassion is a bright Light that illuminates connectedness and love. When you intentionally shift to the Light of compassion, your heart opens by degree and healing is magnified for you and those around you.

One way to help activate a compassionate heart, recommended by the Buddhist teacher Pema Chodron, is to speak the mantra, "Just like me." Look at other people whom you see during the day—family, friends, colleagues, and strangers—and reflect on the fact that,

Just like me, this person has joys and sorrows, and is striving to embrace happiness and avoid suffering. Just like me, this person has losses and disappointments. Just like me, this person wants to feel safe and loved and peaceful. This practice opens your eyes to our similarities and breaks down the barriers to our common humanity.

You can practice "Just like me" on other species as well, such as animals or insects, trees, plants, and flowers, by saying and recognizing the truth of the words, "Just like me." *Just like me, this being is growing, trying to survive, living by instinct, and striving for a pain-free life.*

Compassion is a Light-shift to spiritual healing because it awakens your awareness of the sacred world beyond yourself. There are many ways to develop and encourage your divine compassionate nature to flow. Consider and reflect on the following possible recipients of your compassion:

Compassion for your loved ones who died—for their pain, their struggle, their illness, their fight, their life, their death.

Compassion for others who struggle—with addiction, with illness, with sorrow, with losses, with poverty, with fear, with anxiety, with depression, with shame.

Compassion for animals—for the homeless street dogs and cats, for abused horses, for animals in the wild, for animals losing their natural habitats, for those involved with factory farming.

Compassion for the earth—for the living balance of forests, grasslands, rivers, oceans, and lakes, for the biodiversity that needs nurturing and therefore a keen awareness of recycling, sustainability, reusable resources, and pollution.

Compassion for people who say unhelpful comments—yes, even compassion for the people who say things like "When are you going to move on?" or "When will you be your old self again?" or "You're still grieving?" They simply don't understand. Maybe one day they will but for now, they are confused and say the wrong things.

Compassion for the hurt people who hurt people—perhaps this is the hardest to feel, but it is true that some people who have been hurt and damaged by life, if they aren't emotionally conscious, will perpetuate the chain of pain. They will do what they know and are familiar with—they will continue to pass the torch of anger and hatred.

Compassion is a spiritual state of connection that allows for a deeper healing and lifts you to the spacious perspective of the vertical dimension.

COMPASSION FOR THE SELF

Often, it can feel easier to have compassion for others than to have compassion for oneself. Others deserve compassion, but us? Sometimes we need a reminder—or even a lesson—in how to be *self*-compassionate.

I began working with Ruth when she learned that her son was dying of an aggressive brain cancer. He would likely be dead within a month. Ruth was in her seventies and not in particularly good health herself. She lived in assisted living and wasn't able to be with Roger since he was living in Thailand. Meanwhile, Ruth was no stranger to grief since she had buried a daughter twelve years previously.

Roger was a man of deep faith and wasn't afraid to die. He called his mother daily since they couldn't be together and told her that he was ready to go. His main concern, he told his mother, was that she would be ok. She assured him that she would, though she felt shaken and uncertain.

I saw Ruth weekly as she waited for her son to die. Knowing that he was suffering, she became anxious and irritable as the days unfolded. Finally, Roger crossed over to the other side and Ruth, even in her grief, breathed a sigh of relief that he was out of his pain.

When I saw Ruth the week after he had died, she told me that the *wait* had now turned to *weight*. A feeling of heaviness is a common experience with grief. In fact, the Latin root of grief is *gravare*, which means to make heavy. Yes, grief is oppressively weighty.

Ruth knew what she needed to do now; it's how she got through the death of her daughter. "I'm just going to be the best friend to myself that I can be," she said to me. "I'm going to be gentle and accepting with myself. I'm not going to wish I was happy if I'm not. I know that emotions are fluid and always changing."

Ruth was her own expert, and she had a proven strategy of self-care and self-compassion. Usually, *I'm* explaining this approach to grievers. For most people, they have to be taught how to befriend themselves, how to accept where they are. They need support in asking the question, "What do I most need (or not need) right now?"

LEARNED SELF-COMPASSION

Donald's mother was mentally ill. Well, she hadn't officially been diagnosed, but she often had taken to her bed when Donald was growing up. She had told Donald that she wished she had had a daughter and not a son. He experienced her frequent rages, even wine glasses thrown at the wall. But because humans are complex creatures and because a child is programmed to need the love of his parents, Donald loved his mother dearly.

When Donald was thirty-five years old, his mother died unexpectedly of a heart attack. Donald was grief-stricken. In addition to his sorrow, he also felt guilt and relief and remorse, and a longing for a past that never was.

He was filled with conflicting emotions. On the one hand, he blamed her for many of his adult difficulties and felt that she was a toxic, damaged individual. But on the other hand, he grieved the happy memories he had with her and especially the connection for which he had longed.

Human relationships are messy and complicated. There may be many things that you miss about your loved one but there may be many things that you *don't* miss about your loved one. This is natural. For Donald, part of what he needed was to learn to be gentle with himself, to learn the art of self-compassion. However, at my invitation for him to be kind with himself, he said, "I haven't the slightest idea how to do that."

As children, we are rarely taught the skill of self-compassion. And for most of us it does not come naturally. We might know how to talk kindly and compassionately to a friend but not to ourselves. In fact, one way to start thinking of self-compassion is to ask yourself, *What would I say to a dear friend right now?*

Based on the research of Dr. Kristen Neff, we learn that the essential components of self-compassion are mindfulness, common humanity, and loving kindness. I boil these down to the acronym ACT. ACT stands for

Acknowledge your suffering (mindfulness), Connect with others experiencing this (common humanity), and Talk kindly toward yourself (loving kindness).

I invite you to soothe yourself with self-compassion by engaging the ACT practice when you are experiencing inner conflict with your feelings or thoughts. Begin by putting your hand over your heart. Research shows that this gesture of compassion will stimulate oxytocin. Additionally, if you speak to yourself in the second person, the care circuit part of your brain activates and helps you feel more cared for.

I worked with Donald to come up with the following dialogue for him to say to himself:

1. **A**—Acknowledge your suffering: "Donald, you are feeling so conflicted. You loved your mother but never quite got what you needed from her. She frequently disappointed you and yet, at times, was there for you. It's confusing. This is so rough right now."

2. **C**—Connect to other grievers by remembering you're not alone: "Donald, you're not alone. Many people have messy, complicated relationships and therefore messy, complicated grief."

3. **T**—Talk to yourself kindly: "This is really hard, but you're going to be ok. You deserve

to have your feelings and you deserve to heal. You can look forward to feeling better eventually. Just breathe and take things one moment at a time. You've got this."

Initially, simply ACT as if it is, and you will find that over time, self-compassion will become a natural skill.

Compassion is Spiritual Light in the cracks of your grief.

LIGHT-SHIFT PRACTICES

1—RAIN Meditation

Mindfulness teacher and author Tara Brach says that in all of her years in the field, the RAIN practice is one of her favorite mindfulness techniques for emotional and spiritual healing. The RAIN practice stands for Recognize, Allow, Investigate, and Nurture.

The Practice
When you are feeling especially sad, this practice helps you develop a compassionate awareness of your feelings. Don't judge. Don't criticize. Don't squelch.

Recognize: Name what you are feeling. Research shows that just naming a difficult emotion can reduce its hold on us. Neuroscientists call this "name it to tame it." For example, say, "Yes, this is anger" or "I'm feeling grief; there is intense sorrow and pain."

Allow: Don't reject what you're feeling. Simply let it be without reactivity. Just ALLOW "what is" to be "as it is" in this moment.

Investigate: Check out where you can locate your emotion in the body. This can help to create a sense of curiosity, witnessing, and observing of the sensations in your body. Is there a pit in your stomach? Do you have a clenched jaw, a tight throat, or perhaps an actual ache in your heart area?

Nurture: Bring compassion to this process. Radiate kindness to the part of you having a hard time by putting your hand on any tight body part and saying to yourself something that you might say to a friend: "You're ok. This is so hard. You're going to get through this."

You can enhance this step of nurturing by adding the sequence of "breathe and soften." Breathe into the tight places in your body, soften, and expand what is constricted. Think to yourself, *let me breathe and soften the places that are tight*. This is part of a nurturing, tender, compassionate way to be with yourself.

Think of yourself as a spacious being, expansive enough to hold and honor feelings without being ruled by them. This simple but purposeful practice helps you move from reactivity to receptivity, gently. Mindfulness helps support and heal the broken heart.

2–Metta Meditation of Compassion

I learned the Metta Bhavana practice many years ago at a Buddhist Meditation Center. While it can be difficult to quiet the mind and sit in stillness, the Metta Bhavana, or loving kindness meditation, has several qualities that make it more accessible: (1) It has a specific structure, (2) it feels good, and (3) it gives the mind five specific directions in which to focus.

The Practice

Bring yourself to a comfortable position in a quiet place. Close your eyes and allow yourself to breathe normally. In this meditation you will bring to mind, one at a time, five subjects of your attention. You will imagine white Light cascading over each of them. You can move to the next subject when you are ready or set a meditation timer to ring every one to five minutes and shift to the next subject at the sound of the bell.

To each subject, offer these words:

May you be happy.
May you be healthy.
May you be at peace.
May you be safe from harm.

Visualize the subjects of your attention in the following order:

1. Direct this loving kindness toward yourself.

2. Direct this loving kindness toward someone you dearly love (perhaps your deceased loved one).

3. Direct this loving kindness toward a stranger whom you encountered in the past day or two (the cashier at the grocery store, someone you pass in traffic).

4. Direct this loving kindness toward someone with whom you're having a challenge (this may feel hard to do, but just focus on stating the metta phrases—even if they don't feel genuine yet—as you imagine the person bathed in Light).

5. Direct loving kindness to all beings around the world. Start by imagining Light on your home, on your city, your state or province, your country, the countries around you,

your hemisphere, then wrapping around to
the other side of the globe; then see the globe
as if from outer space, showering all beings
on planet Earth with loving kindness.

3—Journal Prompts

Journaling is a tried-and-true tool for metabolizing
emotion and transforming energy. I have been journaling
for my entire life, ever since I was old enough to write.
It's how I process my experiences. If you have never jour-
naled, you can experiment with a style that suits you.
While some people write in a stream of consciousness,
others prefer guided prompts to shape a reflection.

The Practice
Answer each of the following questions, as you are moved.
Elaborate on the ones that feel the most resonant to you.

- What I learned about grief and loss when I was a
  child was _____.
- What is the hardest part for me about my grief?
- What surprises me about grief?
- What am I learning about myself through this
  process?
- What qualities that my loved one possessed seem
  to be coming through me right now? Or I wish
  were coming through me right now?
- What kind of person do I want to be with my
  grief? With my life?

- When I start to cry, I feel _____.
- When I meet another griever, I want to _____.
- When I think about other people throughout history who have grieved, _____.
- I know I am changing as a result of this loss, and this is how: _____.
- I would like my family to know this about me and my grief: _____.
- When I am most compassionate with myself, I feel _____.
- The word/phrase/mantra of hope and strength that I most want to be my daily guide during this time is _____.

4—Tend a Living Thing

When you're living with loss, you can sometimes spend so much time looking in the rear-view window (at the past, at the deceased) that you forget to look forward (at the future, at the living.) Life is around you—everywhere. See the plants, trees, flowers in your town. See the people and animals around you. Life is still going on and will continue to go on. With your loved one in your heart, you can move forward *with* them. In other words, you don't have to "move on" without your loved one. They're always with you.

You have permission to rejoin the circle of life and be with living things.

The Practice
Intentionally tend to a living thing. It could be a child in your care or a pet or a neighbor or even a houseplant or garden. Notice how you can be present in caretaking. Notice how you put out the food and water, pull the weeds, or bring someone food. Notice how you can make a difference to another living being. Notice how a big smile and a kind word can make a difference during a routine interaction. Open your eyes and decide for a moment, an hour, or a day to show up and be present with the living.

5—Butterfly Hug

The following is a technique developed by Lucina Artigas while working with survivors of Hurricane Pauline in Acapulco, Mexico, in 1998. It is a method of self-soothing known to process traumatic memories and stimulate a calm state. It uses bilateral stimulation to self-administer a healing process.

The Practice
Hold your hands in front of you, so that your palms are facing you. Then, move your right hand to the left and your left hand to your right and link your thumbs together. Now place your hands, with thumbs linked together, onto your upper chest. Start to tap lightly and slowly, right/left, right/left, right/left. Add to this some compassionate words: "I am ok at this moment." "I am not alone even though I feel alone." "All will be well."

"I am enough." "I am grounded." "I am connected to all things."

Experiment with the pressure (light versus firm) and the speed (slow versus fast). Use what feels right to you. Keep tapping until you feel calm and grounded.

CHAPTER 6
FAITH

*Why do you stay in prison when the door
is so wide open?*

—RUMI

Jerusalem stunned me. It wasn't the antiquity, though I loved walking the ancient streets of one of the oldest cities in the world. It wasn't the vibrancy, though I was mesmerized by the smells, sounds, and sights in the old city. It was its sacred pulse, its spirit. There is a powerful spiritual energy to a place that has been sacred to so many generations of people, a holy site to three major Abrahamic religions—Judaism, Christianity, and Islam.

At the Western Wall (remains of the Second Temple begun by Herod the Great, a holy site in Judaism), I felt the energy of Spirit as I saw men and women praying, keening, tucking prayers into the cracks of the wall. I felt all at once the poignancy of centuries of devotion.

At the Church of the Holy Sepulchre (a church built on the traditional site of Jesus's Crucifixion and burial), I wept as the energy of the church and edicule swept me into a higher connection with Spirit. Finally, when I visited the Dome of the Rock, an Islamic shrine, I felt a vortex of sacred energy that made covering my head and slipping off my shoes a natural respectful act.

I was reminded of an experience years before when visiting shrines, temples, and ashrams in India and Nepal when I was mesmerized by the devotional array: prayer wheels, yak butter candles, garlands of marigold flowers, mala beads, statues, and deep resonant chanting. The ancient divine energy was palpable in these sites, sacred to generations of people.

Faith—a confident belief in that which is unseen, a knowing beyond facts or reason. It is a word associated with religious traditions and their commonly held tenets. Indeed, there are many different religious faiths—"windows," so to speak—that look in from different perspectives to the same Light source, Spirit.

Faith, however you experience it, can and does bring comfort to your heart and soul, especially when you're grieving. Whether your faith is a trust in a Higher Power, a deep acceptance of some aspect of the world greater than yourself, or the natural embodiment of the power of human connection and love, your faith will Light your way even down the darkest path.

Soren Kierkegaard said, "Faith sees best in the dark." This line inspired the American President Joe Biden, who is no stranger to the dark night of the soul. He lost a wife and a baby to a car accident in 1972 and later a grown son to brain cancer in 2015. Kierkegaard's quote gave him strength, helped him hold on even when darkness was all that he could see.

Faith gives courage to grievers to keep on living in spite of heart-breaking pain. Consider the example of Corrie ten Boom (1892–1983), a Dutch Christian woman who, with her father and sister, helped Jews escape the Nazis during World War II by hiding them in their home. The three were arrested and sent to the Nazi concentration camp at Ravensbrück, where Corrie's father and sister subsequently died. Corrie survived the terrible ordeal and went on to author *The Hiding Place*, which recounts the story of her family's efforts and how she found hope in God while she was imprisoned at the concentration camp. She was comforted by her faith, which brought her Light in the darkness. She wrote, "There is no pit so deep that God is not deeper still . . . Love is larger than the walls that shut it in."

Even if, at times, your faith falters, dulled by anger, resentment, doubt, or discouragement, keep your heart open to the Light. Allow yourself to rest in the possibility of something more than you currently see or experience.

Faith might have many different looks, but each has the power to lift you out of the darkness. I invite your curiosity and openness to the possibility of your own birthright to faith, your own path to goodness and grace from the mysterious Light of Spirit. The thirteenth-century Sufi mystic Rumi said, *"Stay with it. The wound is the place where the Light enters you."* You have the wound, so be open to the entering Light.

Think of the many dimensions of Light in which you might have faith: faith in the Light of healing and resilience, faith in the Light of the cycle of life, faith in the Light of karma and universal order, faith in the Light of a blessed reunion, and faith in the Light of your alive nature.

FAITH IN HEALING AND RESILIENCE

We are wired for resilience and healing. Just as a cut on your arm eventually heals (even if it leaves a scar), your emotional self is also wired to heal. And just as you might help your wound along with antibiotic cream, stitches, and bandages, likewise you can encourage your emotional self to heal. Not only is emotional healing possible, but just like our bones, our spirit in its healing becomes stronger at the broken places.

Think of how a diamond is formed. Deep within the earth's mantle, carbon atoms are reorganized under extreme high temperatures and pressure. The carbon atoms bond together and create crystals. Then deep-source earth movements deliver the diamonds to the earth's surface. It's a dark and difficult journey, but something beautiful comes out of something quite arduous. We too have the capacity to reform our crushed parts into something new and full of Light.

Challenges create opportunities for transformation and brilliant outcomes. The diamond wouldn't exist without the pressure and heat. Have faith in the possibility of your own creation.

The Vietnamese Buddhist monk, author, teacher, and activist Thich Nhat Hanh shared in his book, *No Mud, No Lotus,* that you can't grow lotus on marble. You need the mud to create the beauty. He taught that you can make good use of your pain when you use it to ultimately create new energies, such as wisdom and compassion. While we are wired for resilience, it helps if you frame your healing as an organic process, like growing a lotus from mud.

FAITH IN THE CYCLE OF LIFE

When I was in high school, I had a poster on my wall of a colorful landscape of New England fall foliage. It was gorgeous. In the bottom right corner of the poster was one single word in calligraphy: DEATH. How prescient that poster now seems. Not only did I grow up to spend twenty-five years living in New England, but I would also become a grief counselor!

I remember that I particularly liked the image because it had never occurred to me that the incandescent beauty of a New England fall was essentially the

death of summer, the death of the leaves that would
shortly fall to the ground, the death of a season. But I
also remember being consoled that even though winter
was sure to follow autumn, spring was sure to follow
winter. In other words, I was consoled by the cycles of
nature.

Even now, the cycles of nature bring me peace: the
caterpillar to butterfly, the seed to tree, the fallen tree
as homes for small creatures, the natural food chain,
the fires that clear out space for new growth, the rainy
seasons, and on and on. There is a rhythm to nature, to
day and night, to full moons and ocean tides. And this
rhythm continues in spite of our stories, our worries, or
our expectations.

I once attended a beautiful Mayan Full Moon
ceremony in Guatemala. Centered around a fire with
symbolic elements, along with cigars whose ash could
divine important messages, I participated in this time-
less ritual of cleansing, releasing, and removing that
which no longer served. We dropped messages, candles,
alcohol, and rose petals into a fire for purification.

While you may not want to engage in a full moon
ceremony every month, some kind of full moon acknowledgement can be a powerful connection to Mother
Earth. Try a moon tradition of lighting a candle, saying
a blessing, or having a special food on this monthly lunar
phase. One of my clients bought a full moon calendar
each year so she could anticipate and honor each monthly
moon with her personalized tradition.

When you note and celebrate earth rhythms the way you would celebrate holidays throughout the year, you start to heighten your connection to earth cycles. Another practice is to become aware of solstices and equinoxes. Solstice ceremonies have been honored by pagan and indigenous cultures for millennia, which traditionally included feasts and sacrifices. Even now, many churches and community groups have ceremonies to acknowledge the solstices, especially the summer solstice (the longest day of the year) and the winter solstice (the shortest day of the year).

Remember that the earth is filled to overflowing with signs of ebb and flow, decay and regeneration, death and rebirth. Intentionally resting in her rhythms and connecting with the web of nature, of which you are a part, will support and nourish you.

FAITH IN KARMA AND UNIVERSAL ORDER

Sometimes faith means believing in something that cannot be proven—such as that there is a design to everything, that there are no accidents, and that everything is as it should be. To believe these things requires the proverbial "leap of faith."

I sat in a chair staring at my own reflection. Fatima was cutting my hair. She wasn't my usual hair stylist, but I was in a new city and needed a change. We were chatting about this and that when suddenly she began to tell me about the death of her sister.

"We were joined at the hip," she told me. "Losing her three years ago was the hardest thing I have ever experienced."

I listened and empathized. "But," she continued, "Our souls contracted for this so even though it's still hard for me, I know it happened exactly as it was supposed to."

This interesting comment sparked a conversation that was calming and comforting to both of us. Fatima shared with me that she had grown up in a Hindi household in which words like reincarnation, karma, and soul contracts are second nature.

When I was studying Tibetan Buddhism, I learned of the belief that souls choose their circumstances before they incarnate—including their parents, their skin color, their nationality, and their socioeconomic station. Souls choose this based on the lessons that they wish to learn and also based on the soul contracts they have with other people in the same lifetime. From this perspective, adversity always has a soul purpose. Those who have faith in this way of seeing life experience an underlying "safety net" of "everything is as it should be," which helps to cultivate peaceful acceptance and resilience.

> All shall be well,
> And All shall be well,
> All manner of things shall be well.
>
> —Julian of Norwich

Even if you don't believe in reincarnation or soul contracts, you can still live with the idea that you'll be okay no matter what. There is more going on than we can see or understand, and opening oneself to that mystery brings a peaceful calm—and a faith—to the process. From this spiritual lens, we can begin to see the path to our own highest healing.

FAITH IN A HEAVENLY REUNION

The translation of "afterlife" in Spanish is "*Mas alla*." But the literal translation of "mas alla" is "more there" or "more beyond." I like the idea of thinking of more, beyond. After all, who really knows for sure? Why not hold out the possibility of a happy reunion?

Audrey was a client who came to see me shortly after her husband Jack passed away. Audrey was in shock because he had died so quickly, so unexpectedly, at the age of seventy-three. She cried every day, longing for her beautiful life with Jack. She and Jack had been together for twenty-five years, a second marriage that brought love and hope into her life when there had been none. Together, they had a blended family of four children, all of whom were inspired by the deep love between Jack and Audrey.

Audrey often asked me, "Do you think I'll be with Jack again, on the other side? I hope so."

I would nod my head and reply, "Well, I don't know for sure, but I believe so. What does your heart tell you?" I used to joke with her that once she got to heaven, whenever that might be, she would need to send me a sign if she was with Jack.

Audrey eventually ended her work with me, ready to reengage with life. Years later, I received an email from Audrey's son giving me the news that Audrey had passed away and inviting me to the funeral.

Audrey was clearly very well loved in her community. The service was touching, poignant. The church was overflowing with a palpable sense that Audrey would be deeply missed. But there was also an explicit expression of hope that Audrey was now reunited with her beloved Jack. There was a relieved acknowledgment that the long wait was over.

As I looked at photos of the two of them during the reception, my heart was warmed. When I went back to my car after the reception, I opened my door and looked down. There, to my surprise, I discovered a white feather on my car seat.

I blinked twice. I looked around—was my car window down, had someone placed this here? Had my car been locked? Wait, what?

I simply smiled. I knew it was Audrey's sign to me. I was sure of it. She and Jack were together again.

While many grievers have faith that there will be a reunion on the other side, not Joe. Joe found his own spiritual path to reunion, to peace. When Joe lost his beloved wife of forty-six years, he was crushed. While he was adamant that he didn't believe he would see Rosa on the other side, it didn't trouble him. He told me that his job was to keep her alive in his memory and in the memory of his children, his stepchildren, and his grandchildren. "That's the only eternity I believe in," he said. "Alive in the hearts of those who remember."

Joe had faith in the continuity of her spirit. He told me that her energy was in the tree that took nourishment from her ashes scattered at its base. "Her spirit is in the natural world," he said, "complete in its cycle of ashes to ashes, dust to dust."

FAITH IN YOUR ALIVENESS

Something more is coming. You are still the one left on planet Earth. Be curious and open to finding the reason why. They say that after a door closes, somewhere else a door opens. Will you recognize that open door, your reason for still being alive?

Rumi said:

> *Sorrow prepares you for joy. It violently sweeps*
> *everything out of your house, so that new joy*

can find space to enter. It shakes the yellow
leaves from the bough of your heart, so that
fresh, green leaves can grow in their place. It
pulls up the rotten roots, so that new roots
hidden beneath have room to grow.

Chadwick Boseman, an American actor and producer who died in 2020 of colon cancer, gave a commencement address at Howard University, his alma mater. He said, "Purpose is an essential element of you. It is the reason you are on the planet at this particular time in history. Your very existence is wrapped up in the things you are here to fulfill."

The griever's journey is about feeling pain, mourning deeply, focusing on healing, reengaging with life, and making meaning. Remember that you are a spiritual being having a human experience. You might ask yourself, "What does life expect of me? What is life asking of me?"

Perhaps you don't know yet. That's fine. Have faith in your aliveness and ask for guidance. It can feel as if you're in the hallway between rooms and you're not sure what's behind the door just ahead of you. Get comfortable in the hallway and take all the time you need. But when you're ready and willing, when you can see your inner compass for direction, walk up to the new doorway and knock. It opens to a new world of possibility and transcendence.

Faith is Spiritual Light in the cracks of your grief.

LIGHT-SHIFT PRACTICES

1—Cycle Syllables

This quick and simple practice, from the Hindu tradition, uses your fingers and a few syllables to bring the entire cycle of life and death into your hands. The following Sanskrit syllables—SA, TA, NA, MA—signify "birth," "life," "destruction," "regeneration."

They speak to faith and acceptance in the cycles of life.

The Practice

While you repeat the syllables SA, TA, NA, MA, touch the following fingers of each hand to your thumb.

Thumb to pointer finger, say SA (sah).

Thumb to middle finger, say TA (tah).

Thumb to ring finger, say NA (nah).

Thumb to pinky finger, say MA (mah).

Repeat this sequence six times, using both hands simultaneously.

> For the first two rounds, say the syllables out loud.

> For the second two rounds, say the syllables in a whisper.

> For the final two rounds, think the syllables silently within your own head.

Breathe deeply and notice the feeling of peacefulness settling over you.

2—Central Channel Breath

I learned about this breathing technique from Sue Morter's work described in her book, *The Energy Codes*. It has to do with connecting—through your breath—to a column of energy that runs between the heavens and the earth, through your body. Whatever your concept of spiritual Light. your faith is strengthened when you visualize your connection to it.

The Practice
Sit or stand comfortably.

Inhale deeply, and as you inhale, visualize breathing energy (or Light) up from the earth, through the soles of your feet, filling your body. Then, exhale deeply, visualizing shimmering energy (or Light) out through the top of your head, toward the sky.

Next, reverse direction. Inhale deeply, drawing energy (or Light) from the sky, from the vast heavens, the Light cascading down through the crown of your head, filling your body. Then, exhale deeply, sending energy (or Light) shooting down through your feet toward the earth, imagining energy going straight down to the center of the earth.

Engage in this "central channel breathing" for a few more cycles of breath. Feel your body as a conduit of energy connecting you to heaven and earth.

To add even more power to this grounding breath, squeeze the pelvic bowl of your body. Do this by contracting your muscles as if you were trying to stop the flow of urine midstream. This contraction concentrates energy at the tip of your spine, your root chakra. This fifteenth-century yogic technique, known as mula bandha, creates a root lock that grounds the core of the body.

Keep breathing and imagining Light energy flowing through you from heaven to earth and back again. Notice if and/or how it feels differently to you when you add the mula bandha element to the breath.

3—Heaven Rushing In

Donna Eden, healer and Energy medicine teacher, describes the Radiant Circuits as one of the nine energy systems in the body that, when activated, initiates a feeling of wonder, happiness, and joy. In ancient

Chinese medicine, this subtle energy is known as Strange Flows or Extraordinary Vessels and is responsible for supporting the meridians (the energy channels that move through the body).

This simple practice, a part of Donna Eden's Radiant Circuit routine, utilizes intentional awareness of Light in the sky to shift and increase positive energy in your body. It enhances feelings of expansion and connection to all that is, and thus energizes your capacity for transcendence.

The Practice

While you are outside, or if you can look outside a window, look up to the Light and extend your arms wide, up and open, to the sky, to the heavens. Say, "I receive sun and Light, love and life, and all good things in this world and beyond." Then, scoop it all in by bringing your hands to your heart. They say that there is a vortex there, in your heart chakra, that is filled with goodness as heaven rushes in. If you feel like you'd like a little more goodness, repeat the process.

4—Things are Looking Up

Notice how your eyes mostly stay on a horizontal plane during an average day. Yes, we sometimes look up and we sometimes look down, but we spend a shocking amount of time looking right in front of us (driving, sitting in front of computers, watching TV, playing video games, talking with the person across from us).

Faith is a willingness to see what is not right in front of you. Get your eyes working vertically. Let them take you to the vertical dimension of existence.

The Practice
Breathe. Inhale and move your eyes up, looking toward the ceiling or the sky. Stretch your eyes. Then, exhale and move your eyes to the right and all the way down, toward the ground. Imagine the vast vertical energy from the sky to the depth of the earth. Now, move your eyes left and back up toward the sky.

Do this vertical eye stretch five to ten times, giving your eyes a chance to exercise the muscles.

When you're done stretching your eyes, rest by looking up. Go outside or look out a window to the sky if you're able and spend some time watching the clouds, observing the colors, seeking the stars. If you're not able to go or look outside, then take a few minutes to observe the ceiling, its textures and colors. Looking up has a way of literally and metaphorically taking you out of yourself.

5—Prayer Candle
Lighting a candle is known the world over as a sacred ritual. Often there is an area in Catholic or Episcopal churches to specifically light candles on behalf of ill or deceased individuals. In Hindu temples, lighting a candle represents burning away impurities. And for

Tibetan Buddhists, lighting a yak butter lamp helps to focus the mind and aid meditation.

A candle is a symbolic means to bring Light into darkness, a visual reminder of faith and the importance of Light-shifting.

The Practice

Light a candle and connect to your faith through silence, through a mantra, or through a prayer.

You can make up your own prayer. Or simply say, "Thank you." As Meister Eckhart, the thirteenth-century German theologian said, "If the only prayer you ever say in your entire life is thank you, it will be enough."

Or try saying "The Serenity Prayer":

> *Grant me the strength to accept the things I*
> *cannot change,*
> *the courage to change the things I can,*
> *and the wisdom to know the difference.*

Or try the "A Course in Miracles" prayer:

> *Where would you have me go?*
> *What would you have me do?*
> *What would you have me say?*
> *And to whom?*

You might ask for a blessing on your loved one, ask for

a blessing on yourself, or pray for the well-being of all beings who know love and loss.

Watch the center of the flame of your candle. Take a pause to center yourself and, after your prayers, to sit in silence. Notice how the silence beckons stillness. Allow yourself to simply BE, a vertical act in and of itself.

After what feels like a comfortable amount of time for you, blow out your candle deliberately and mindfully watch the smoke circle up to the heavens, lifting your prayers and well wishes to a different dimension.

May this practice lift you to a higher place, helping to relax your ego and connect with Spirit, of which you are an integral part.

PART 3:

A HIGHER HEALING

Goodbyes are only for those who love with their eyes. Because for those who love with heart and soul there is no such thing as separation.

—RUMI

A Hindu master noticed that his apprentice complained daily about his lack of spiritual progress. So, one morning, the master decided to offer his apprentice a new lesson, and he sent the young man for some salt. When the apprentice returned, the master instructed the impatient young man to put a handful of salt in a glass of water and then to drink it.

"How does it taste?" the master asked.

"Bitter," sputtered the apprentice.

The two walked in silence to a nearby lake. The

master asked the young man to mix a handful of salt in the lake. When the apprentice had finished stirring salt into the water, the old man said, "Now drink from the lake."

The young man did so and then the master asked, "How does it taste?"

"Fresh," noted the apprentice.

"Do you taste the salt?" asked the master.

"No," said the young man.

At this, the master took the hands of this serious young man, offering his reflection, "The pain of life is pure salt; no more, no less. The amount of pain in life remains the same. But the bitterness we taste depends on the container we put the pain in. Stop being a glass. Become a lake."

I have always loved this story because it points to the power of expansion. When you allow yourself to expand to the vertical dimension of your life (a bigger container for the salt), you are able to honor and tolerate the pain of loss within the vast expanse of love. While loss is your constant companion, you have the opportunity to hold it in an ever-larger container. As we know, grief doesn't end, but your relationship with it can change.

Remember this image from earlier in the book? The grief in your life doesn't necessarily go away but it becomes less intense as you expand around it.

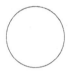

LIFE
BEFORE LOSS

LIFE
WITH LOSS

LIFE AFTER LOSS
EXPANDED

As you toggle between the "being with" your grief and "looking up" from your grief, you cultivate the four divine experiences: dwelling in **love**, focusing on **connection**, initiating **compassion**, and deepening your **faith**. However, there is an experience that deepens your relationship to your loved one and takes you even higher, something that can occur initially but usually develops over the arc of time: **transcendence**. Transcending is finding and living with a purpose. It is an experience that brings meaning to your life and to your loved one's death.

Transcendence is the intentional act of taking grief and repurposing it to its highest potential. When you see from a higher vantage point, things look and feel different. As your vista expands, you begin to make choices based on your new insights. Yes, the grief is still there, but now it's a part of an expanding world of love, connection, compassion, and faith.

In Chinese, the character for "crisis" implies both hardship and growth. The symbol is comprised of two characters, the first meaning "dangerous" and the second meaning "point of change." So too, in the "crisis" of grief, you have a choice point to open to opportunity instead of dwelling in danger.

Transcendence is a Light-shift from the feeling that loss is happening TO you, and instead that loss is happening FOR you. And why? It's happening for you to grow, to give, to reach out, to touch, to change things, to make a difference, to find a purpose, and to honor your loved one.

This final chapter looks at how you can choose Transcendence at any point in your process. It might happen early on your journey, or it may emerge over time. I like to think of sea glass as yet another metaphor for conceptualizing the path to transcendence. The early stages of grief are like the sharp shards of glass that make their way to the sea. As you move from Shock to Disorganization to Reconstruction, as you live with Synthesis and choose the four divine experiences (Love, Connection, Compassion, Faith), the glass is being tumbled, changed, worn, smoothed by sand and salt and pounding waves. Over time, it becomes something beautiful, something luminous.

A widow client in the early stage of grief once told me that she had "no choice" but to survive. Over time, she came to understand that while there was no choice that her loved one had died, she actually had many, many choices with her grief. Every griever has the choice to feel their feelings or repress them, a choice to engage with life or withdraw, a choice to focus on what you had or on what you lost, a choice to Light-shift or not. You get to *choose* how you want to be with your grief.

When, over time, you begin to choose Transcendence, you collect the shards of your grief and transform them, like sea glass, into frosted, prized pieces, the foundation for beautiful art.

It's never too late. You can accept the invitation to meaning and purpose offered by grief no matter how many years have gone by.

CHAPTER 7

TRANSCENDENCE

The only lasting beauty
is the beauty of the heart.

—RUMI

Viktor Frankl wrote, "Everything can be taken from a man but one thing: the last of the human freedoms—to choose one's attitude in any given set of circumstances, to choose one's own way." Victor should know since he was a survivor of the Second World War Holocaust.

Before the war, Victor was a successful Jewish neurologist and psychiatrist living in Vienna with his new wife. In 1942, he had everything taken from him—his home, his family, his personal possessions, his work. He was sent to a series of concentration camps where he was forced to endure unspeakable horrors. His wife and parents and brother all died in the camps. Somehow,

Victor survived, buoyed by his belief in the power of human hope and the will to meaning.

Even before the war, Victor believed that purpose matters. People who have a purpose are healthier, live longer, and have a higher sense of well-being. After the war, he was even more convinced of this truth. He frequently quoted the German philosopher Nietzsche, who said, "Whoever has a *why* to live can bear almost any *how*."

Victor also wrote, "If we can't change our fate, at least we can accept it, adapt, and possibly undergo inner growth even in the midst of troubles." He went on to summarize that there are three primary ways to find a sense of purpose in life: (1) Through the dignity of facing a situation that cannot be changed (such as death or grief); (2) through love; and (3) through outward actions, emphasizing that the door to meaning opens outward away from self-interests.

He is most famous for his 1946 book *Man's Search for Meaning.* However, three of his post-war public lectures, which were delivered in Vienna in 1946 just nine months after he was liberated from a labor camp, have been translated into English and collected into a book called *Yes to Life: In Spite of Everything.*

He was an alchemist, really, who believed in transforming something terrible into something better. Alchemy, the mysterious medieval chemical science, worked to transmute base metals into gold. Now the idea of alchemy is one of taking what you have, however challenging, and working to transmute it into something positive, something meaningful. Frankl's life work is a testimony to this possibility and a beacon of inspiration for each of us.

REACHING OUT

Claude was a sixty-three-year-old man who was my client for four years. After his only child died of a drug overdose, he was devastated. He was beyond devastated, actually. After two decades of trying to help his daughter but watching her spin out of control—from rehab to rehab, from prison to prostitution—Claude let go. He adopted a "tough love" approach and refused to give her money or shelter. And suddenly, amazingly, things started to turn around. But just when it seemed like his daughter was getting better, she died of a drug overdose.

Claude was inconsolable. He felt guilty, remorseful, responsible—all of it. He was riddled with "if onlys" and "what if I had said yes instead of no?" He felt suicidal, telling me that he had nothing to live for and prayed every day for God to take him. It seemed to him that there was nothing left.

I validated his experience, normalized his pain and regret, and helped him tolerate his pain. For two years, it seemed, there was little progress. But over time, the extreme pain was less intense, and his episodes of depression were less frequent. He began to realize that God wasn't going to take him, at least not yet.

One day he told me, "If I'm going to be alive, I might as well do something useful." I encouraged him and told him about Viktor Frankl's work. He began to reflect on the seeds of purpose in his life.

One thing led to another, and Claude came to realize an intense desire to help kids struggling with addiction and the parents who loved them. He put his community service skills to use and began speaking in local schools and at PTA meetings. He volunteered in a rehab center. He reached out to parents whose kids were battling the battle that he knew only too well. And he did all of this in honor of his daughter.

In other words, he framed his work intentionally as a direct outcome of his pain and his grief. He said, "I do this work because of my daughter, for my daughter, in honor of my daughter." And the people he helped as a result were helped because of her experience and her life. Her life rippled outward, touching other lives, and on and on. Claude's life rippled outward. Tragedy alchemized to meaning.

Did Claude's pain completely disappear? Of course not. But his pain became one of the threads in the fabric of his larger mission. He stopped asking God to take him and instead asked God for more time so he could keep making a difference. He hadn't been able to save his daughter's life, but he could make meaning out of his loss by helping to save the lives of others.

FINDING YOUR MITZVAH

Years ago, Dr. Sol Gordon, a clinical psychologist, introduced the idea of "mitzvah therapy." In the Jewish tradition, a mitzvah is a good deed that is offered without any expectation of thanks. It's a holy obligation. In working with clients, Dr. Gordon suggested that they take the focus off of themselves and their own troubles and instead channel their energy into offering mitzvahs in the world. Mitzvah is all about doing good.

Examples of mitzvahs might be starting a foundation or business, or committing to a volunteer position, or using one of your skills to help others. The point is to allow your pain to motivate you toward something positive.

Janice, a fifty-five-year-old seamstress and a widow, uses her sewing skills to help other grievers. She specializes in making memorial quilts, handcrafted quilts of all sizes made with the unique clothes of the client's departed loved one. She keeps her prices relatively low, thus making it affordable for as many people as possible. She told me, "I love knowing that grievers will be wrapped in love, literally in the clothes of their loved ones."

She occasionally branches out to decorative pillows and even teddy bears, all made from the clothes of grievers' loved ones. "I love when people get their item and they're just blown away seeing the creation that I've made, which is so intimate, since it has special shirts, or dresses or ties that they remember so fondly," she says.

And since she's a widow, she gets it. She never imagined that she would start this labor of love, which connects her to other bereaved individuals, but for her, it is a mitzvah that continues to make meaning from her own loss.

HELPING THE BEREAVED

Helping other bereaved individuals is, in fact, a quite natural form of Transcendence. After all, grievers understand loss from the inside out and are uniquely educated and qualified to help other grievers.

For some, this service is informal—such as reaching out to friends, or even strangers, who you know are dealing with loss. Annie, a widow who was elderly and bedridden, decided that she wanted to send condolence letters the old-fashioned way—with actual cards. Through her church and through friends of friends, she connected with people who had suffered recent losses. She felt it was her mission to send condolence cards every week, "just to let them know that someone understands and cares."

Or, reaching out can also be more formal—such as becoming a trained hospice or hospital volunteer or bereavement group facilitator. Many people find that they want to give back through the organizations that were the most helpful to them when they were going through their loved ones' illness and/or dying process.

I have seen grievers become active in both hospice groups and grief groups. My client Arthur became so active in the grief organization, The Compassionate Friends (a national resource for bereaved parents), that he took on a leadership role in organizing their annual national conference.

For others, it means a complete career change. Gina was best friends with her wife, her partner. In fact, as an only child to an only child single mom, Gina didn't grow up with much family—no dad, no siblings, no aunts or uncles, no cousins. Laura became Gina's family, her everything. They were inseparable and in love for thirty-eight years.

When Laura was killed by a drunk driver, Gina was inconsolable. It felt as if the center of her world evaporated. Gina allowed herself to grieve but felt very alone in it. While grief is universal and ubiquitous, she felt misunderstood as she suffered her invisible wound. So, she sought involvement in a community of people who might understand her experience: Widow Club, a community which offers several in-person retreats per year.

While she wanted to be around people who understood, she soon discovered that the LGBTQ community was underrepresented. She took it upon herself to become a voice for deepening the understanding of that disenfranchised group. It's one thing to lose your spouse, but it's another thing to have people believe that your grief is somehow "less than" because you don't fit the hetero-cultural norm.

Gina found a mission to help people understand that love is the core essence of grief. Her message was that the grief journey is about love, loss, and healing, not about race, gender, or socioeconomic background.

Gina ended up leaving her career as a paralegal to work full time with Widow Club. She became passionate about helping all grievers feel validated and included.

Grief is the great equalizer, and she wanted to make sure that no widow or widower ever felt judged for the depth of their grief or the depth of their love.

CARRYING ON THE LEGACY

Carrying on the legacy means to complete something that your loved one started. This is an example of a Light-shift that leads to greater meaning. In chapter 5 on Connection, I offered the example of the father who walked the ancient pilgrimage known as "El Camino" in Spain since his son hadn't been able to complete that journey.

Another example is Mitchell Denburg, who spent two years fighting to cure his wife, Lissie Habie, after she was diagnosed with a brain tumor. Lissie was an artist in Guatemala. Upon facing her imminent death, she asked her husband, "Please don't leave my art in boxes in a closet. Let it be seen."

After her death, he opened a visual-arts cultural space with her art as a centerpiece in the permanent collection. In addition to making sure that her art was seen, he began to foster the careers of local Guatemalan artists. His gallery, La Nueva Fábrica, sponsors an artist-in-residency program, exhibitions, community events, and fundraisers to support artists.

He told me that he wanted to make Lissie proud of him, every day. Clearly, he has achieved that. In shifting to the Light of her legacy, he has extended her impact and enriched the lives of many.

TOUCHING LIVES

Transcendence can be an ongoing project, a one-time event, a changing passion, or a recurring tradition. Sometimes a special day can become a reason to find a transcendent response. A birthday, wedding anniversary, or angelversary (another name for the anniversary of the death day) are perfect days to honor your loved one with purpose.

For example, Steve is a man who donates money every year in honor of his daughter. He always selects a grassroots organization that will take his donation and personally apply it to needy families with children. Each year, from a different country, he receives personalized photographs of small children who hold up hand-colored signs that say, "In memory of Jacqui."

He told me, "I can't describe how it feels to see those little children knowing that Jacqui is the reason they're receiving help. It warms my heart . . . and for years, I didn't think that my heart would ever feel warmth again." Framing his actions as "on her behalf," gives him a purpose. "Helping is healing," he says.

Transcendence doesn't bring your loved one back or eliminate pain, but it does extend their reach, their impact, and their meaning beyond you and out into the world. Transcendence is the bigger container—the expanded dimension—for grief, that which makes the salt taste less bitter.

GETTING AWAY FROM IT ALL

It may be that you have come to a place where transcendence sounds like a good idea, but you just aren't sure what to do or how to do it. Maybe you have the willingness but not the inspiration. For many, the inspiration, the Light of transcendence shines through in moments of stillness. One suggestion I have, for the purpose of giving yourself time to sit with stillness, is to go on a retreat. A change of scenery with the time to be quiet, without other responsibilities, can be a big game changer.

There are many possibilities for retreat. A formal retreat can last a day or a week; it might be organized through a church or monastery, a meditation center or yoga studio. You could also organize your own respite at the beach, by a lake, or in the mountains. The idea is to leave your home and enter an environment that will cultivate your interior landscape (your inscape). This wouldn't be an ordinary vacation or even a weekend at your favorite hotel; the idea is to have the intention of being with Spirit. You might sit in silence, walk a labyrinth, stretch your body, or be with others on their journey of self-discovery. Retreats offer the opportunity for deep interior listening, for soul spaciousness, and for awareness of your inner compass. They offer you an opportunity to discern your next direction.

Even if a spiritual retreat is not available to you right now, file away the idea for your future. It might be the key to your door to transformation.

GRIEF AND GRATITUDE

Lastly, there is one more natural aspect of transcendence that is important to reflect upon—gratitude. Transcendence itself is an act of gratitude. While you aren't grateful for the death, you cultivate gratitude for what was, gratitude for what can be, and gratitude for what exists in this moment. On your quest to make meaning out of loss, the new actions/work/relationships and possibilities that you've created only exist now *because* of the loss of your loved one. These things didn't exist before, so you can be grateful for the new things that have emerged from your loved one's life and death.

The word transcendence comes from the Latin prefix *trans*, meaning "beyond," and *scandare*, meaning "to climb up." You go upward, vertically, to a higher place beyond limitations, and in that place, you have a macro view that gives you perspective on the whole. From that vantage point, you can see a big picture and notice the patterns; you can nurture your alchemical inner transformation and dial into gratitude.

One rich aspect of gratitude is that it builds on itself. Terry told me after her twin sister's death from a sudden heart attack, "I live life now, for my sister. She's not here so I take it upon myself to appreciate this life . . . for my sake and for her sake. My gratitude for being alive is a chance to feel connected to my sister." She continued, "Sometimes it's as if I am seeing the world through my sister's eyes and she is smiling."

The death of your loved one has led you to places and emotions and growth and experiences where you never would have gone otherwise. Notice how, when, and where you can be grateful for these experiences. Examples could include:

- gratitude for having loved and been loved
- gratitude for the love that still lives in your heart
- gratitude for sweet memories
- gratitude for good medical care
- gratitude for emergency personnel
- gratitude for the friends and family who offered support
- gratitude for grief support services
- gratitude for the people you've met because of your grief
- gratitude for the compassion you've developed

- gratitude that you can continue to connect with your loved one
- gratitude that your faith has broadened
- gratitude that you no longer fear death
- gratitude for signs from the beyond
- gratitude for angels in your life
- gratitude for nature and beauty
- gratitude that you have found ways to make meaning
- gratitude that you transformed your grief into purpose
- gratitude that you are still here growing
- gratitude that there are still many blessings in your life
- gratitude that you're on a path to higher healing

You don't forget that you loved someone who left the planet. You don't forget that they're still with you in some form. Carla told me that usually bereaved parents hate the innocuous question, "How many kids do you have?" But she loves the question. She answers, "I have a daughter who is twenty-eight and is an engineer in Denver, and I have a Spirit son who will be forever twelve years old." She goes on to emphasize how grateful she was to be his mom and how she honors his memory every day through her actions and words. Then she cautions her listener to remember that life is precious, often brief, and you shouldn't waste your time here.

As the Buddhist spiritual teacher Pema Chodron said, "Everything in life has the potential to either wake us up or put us back to sleep." Let grief wake you up. Let it teach you about gratitude and all the ways we can open to deeper experiences of love.

Transcendence is Spiritual Light in the cracks of your grief.

LIGHT-SHIFT PRACTICES

1—Gratitude Magnet

Gratitude is a direct path to inner peace and happiness. Practicing gratitude with intention creates an upward spiral of consciousness and well-being. It helps you feel more blessed, content, loving, and peaceful. In other words, gratitude generates *more* gratitude.

The Practice

This practice has three options, each more challenging. Choose one or practice with all three.

> **Foundation option**—notice three things from your day for which you are grateful. This is possible even on a day when you are overcome with sadness. Notice the sky, the air, hot water,

air-conditioning. Notice grass, flowers, your ability to breathe. Say out loud, "I give thanks for . . ." Take a moment with each one and really feel it. Savor each as a gift.

More challenging option—recall a specific memory with your loved one and be grateful that you had that experience with them. Take a moment to remember and feel what that moment was like. It's okay if sadness and gratitude are mixed—you can hold them both together. But for this exercise, Light-shift your attention to the gratitude and say, "I'm so grateful that . . ." Savor the gift of it.

Most challenging option—give thanks for what your grief is teaching you and for where it's leading you. This is challenging because, of course, you would always rather have your loved one present and forgo any sort of positive outcome of your grief. But given that you are where you are and grief is in your life, what can you appreciate about it? Say out loud, "Thank you grief for teaching me about . . . and helping me grow in this way . . . or leading me in this direction . . ." Savor the gifts that grow out of loss.

2—Legacy Haiku

A haiku is a short poetic form originating in Japan in the seventeenth century as a reaction to long and elaborate poetic traditions. It wasn't known by the name haiku until the nineteenth century. It consists of three lines in a predictable pattern of five syllables, seven syllables, five syllables. Originally, the art form focused on nature and the seasons, but the modern haiku can be about any topic.

Using a simple structure to focus and distill your thoughts and feelings can help you express and metabolize your grief. Expressing your feelings in an art form is a vertical experience in which you elevate energy to a higher level.

The Practice
Write one or more haiku poems. Here are some prompts that might help you get started:

- The legacy left by your loved one.
- Who do you want to be with your grief?
- How do you want to make your grief meaningful?
- What do you imagine your loved one would say about your grieving process?
- What beauty can you share with your loved one?

Here are some examples:

Buttermilk biscuits
Big Mama's southern cooking
Food translates to love

A seed of pain grows
Beyond its confines to more
Plant turns toward light

Dark cloud over me
I do not know where to turn
Flower at my feet

Where, where did she go?
Will I ever get a sign?
Blue bird on the porch

3—Random Acts of Kindness

One of my clients, Serena, was searching for a way to honor her husband on the first angelversary. Another widow friend of hers suggested doing a Random Act of Kindness in honor of Greg. She was so touched by the idea that she took it even further: she had cards printed up that included Greg's photo, a brief bio, and the words, "You're the recipient of this Random Act of Kindness in honor of Greg's life. Please pay it forward in his honor."

In this way, she told me, more Random Acts of Kindness would be generated—all in honor of Greg. For her, she went out to eat and paid the bill of the couple next to her in the restaurant. She told the waitress, "After I leave, when they ask for the bill, just tell them that the bill was paid by Greg and then give them this card."

Serena decided that she would honor Greg every year on his angelversary, on his birthday, at Christmas time, and on their wedding anniversary. Days that might be painful triggers could also become days of spreading good energy, love, and kindness. The loss of Greg—the love for Greg—became the momentum for a movement toward kindness.

The Practice

Come up with your own brand of a Random Act of Kindness. You don't have to print cards with your loved one's image, but you can know that you're doing it in their honor. Some examples: pay a bill for someone, pay the toll for the car behind you, send anonymous flowers to a friend, drop off donuts at an office or library, drop coins outside of stores, leave stones with happy words on them in public places, send a card to someone who is sick or struggling in some way, leave food out for homeless animals, donate books to a preschool or daycare center, leave "love notes" in library books for a reader to find, or leave "love notes" in public places such as on drug store or grocery shelves (such as "You're amazing," or "You're loved," or "You can do it," or "You've got this," or "Spread kindness," or "Share your Light"). Do any one of these things—or your own idea—in honor of your loved one. Their impact extends through you.

4—Open Heart Posture

Having an open heart increases the likelihood of creating transcendence in your life. When you're experiencing a shattered and aching heart, it's useful to spend some time working to open your heart chakra.

The chakra system, from the ancient yogic tradition in India, is an energy system of seven wheels, or vortexes, running from the base of your spine to the crown of your head. These energy centers regulate your prana, or life force. Keeping your chakras open and balanced keeps you healthy in all ways.

Similarly, in the Chinese tradition of acupuncture and acupressure, there is a point called the ming men point, which is known as the gate to life's vitality. Pressing on the ming men point not only revitalizes energy but forces your body to open up the chest cavity, thereby giving space and energy to the heart chakra.

The following practice builds on both the Indian and Chinese medical traditions to soothe and calm your heart so that it will soften into compassion for yourself and others.

The Practice

You can locate the ming men point on your back by drawing an imaginary line directly from your belly button through your body to your back. Ming men means "Gate of Life" or "Gate of Destiny" and is a strengthening point. First, rub your palms together and then bring your hands around to your lower back, using your fingertips to cover the ming men point. This naturally pulls your arms backward, bringing your shoulder blades together. As you lift and open the chest cavity, you also open up energy for your heart chakra.

For added emphasis lift your chin up and gaze toward the heavens, receiving every blessing. Breathe low and deeply for several slow breath cycles, feeling your rib cage expand and your heart area open.

5—Lullaby Chants

We can learn deep truths from many different religious traditions. Chanting is a hypnotic repetition of a word or phrase, often to a singsong tone, which has been used across multiple cultures and eras. Gregorian chants were popular during the ninth and tenth centuries in western and central Europe in the Roman Catholic Church. Named after St. Gregory I, a Pope in the late sixth century, Gregorian chants found a popular resurgence in the twentieth century amongst monastic men and women in religious orders.

With roots in the Hindu vedic tradition, kirtans are a call-and-response chant, usually set to music, in which a legend is described or spiritual ideas are expressed. Higher states of consciousness are induced with the lilting, lullaby patterns of these chants.

Tribal cultures, such as Native American or African, often have chants with a drum accompaniment and communal dancing, often around a sacred fire. Ancient cultures knew that chanting transcends the senses and takes us to a place beyond time and space. When we dwell in this hypnotic state, we open up access to future possibilities.

The Practice

In the Hindu tradition, a popular chant is "Om Namah Shivaya." This means "Universal Consciousness is One." Try chanting this phrase over and over again. You might want to look on YouTube to listen to multiple versions of this chant set to music. Or simply chant the sound "Om," if that is more comfortable.

You could also try "Yeha-Noha," which is from the Navajo Indian tradition. This means "wishes of happiness and prosperity."

Or you could simply chant, "Glory, Alleluia" from the Judeo-Christian tradition.

Listen to sacred chants from around the world and let yourself be lulled into a higher state of being. See which ones resonate the most for you.

RECLAIMING LIFE

Your heart is the size of an ocean.
Go find yourself in its hidden depths.

—*RUMI*

For many years, each of my psychotherapy sessions has begun in the same way: with stillness and a bell. It's a transition ritual—a brief mindfulness meditation to help the client transition from their day and become present in the moment, to help them "arrive." It is always a welcome pause, a moment of peace.

We close our eyes, and I say, "Resting into now, coming to center. Let yourself BE with what is, as it is, in this moment in time, inviting curiosity and openness toward whatever needs to arise. When you hear the sound of the bell, let the tone calm you, ground you, and take you deeper and deeper within, to a place of inner spaciousness. Breathe in the bell." Then I ring a Tibetan singing bowl three times and we listen to the sound. Ding. Ding. Ding.

As the final sound resonates, I think to myself: *Source Energy, Make me an instrument of Divine Love and Light.* This brief pause is a win-win: a transition ritual for the client and a critical moment for me to align with the vertical.

I find that my own spiritual framework has been strengthened by my work. Without my faith, I would have burned out and lost hope, both personally and professionally, a long time ago. I fervently believe that Spirit is gracious and good, lovingly supporting both me and my clients.

My own verticality has given me the strength to bear witness to unspeakable pain and tragic loss. I trust that when people are broken open, powerful transformations are possible. And I believe that even those who are lost in the darkness can eventually find their way to Light.

Sometimes people ask me, "Isn't it depressing to work with grievers and be surrounded by so much sadness?"

Yes, there are times when the work breaks my heart. So many years of loss, of tears to witness, of sorrow on my shoulders. But at the same time, I am filled with hope. I witness the beauty of resilience, love, and strength. As Ernest Hemingway said, "The world breaks everyone and afterward many are strong at the broken places." And I would say that many are even *golden* at the broken places.

Doing this work reminds me of my own mortality and the impermanence of life. My work reminds me that nothing is guaranteed. Every day I have an invitation to savor my blessings and not take things for granted. This awareness blows the dust off of life, allowing me to see clearly the gifts of the present moment. This moment, now, is all that we ever have.

Lastly, doing this work for three decades has, for me, crystallized the perspective that love is eternal, life is vast, and that what we see on planet Earth is only a small part of a larger picture. There is an expansive design to our growth and our experiences. We simply need to let Spirit lift us up and root us down so that we know we are not alone.

A MATTER OF LIFE AND DEATH

I have always loved the Thornton Wilder 1938 play *Our Town*, a classic whose main themes are the inevitability of death and the sweet gift of life. I was cast in the role of Mrs. Webb in high school and so remember the play with intimate fondness. One of the main characters, Emily, is a young girl who marries her high school sweetheart George. However, by the beginning of Act 3, Emily has recently died in childbirth. Act 3 is about her spirit revisiting a day in her life, witnessing herself as she lived.

Emily enters the scene of her twelfth birthday and notices how everyone is just going about the morning, taking it all for granted. She wants to shout to her mama that in fourteen years she, Emily, will marry George and die in childbirth.

Emily wishes that her mother would *really* look at her, as a twelve-year-old, and hug her, knowing that these things are in the future. She watches how no one actually sees each other against the backdrop of impermanence. She is troubled by what she views as the blindness—the ignorance—of everyday living.

It eventually becomes too poignant and too painful to watch. Emily asks to leave, saying goodbye to all the details of life, and proclaiming, "Oh earth, you're too wonderful for anybody to realize you." She asks the narrator if anyone ever realizes the preciousness of life while they live it. He answers, "The saints and poets, maybe—they do some."

It's a wonderful life, even with loss and heartbreak and despair. You are still here for a reason. And while you may not know why at the moment, you are still here. You have time to spend, to use, to wake up to the vertical dimension in your precious life.

Let this book be your invitation to smooth the sharp edges of your grief, to shift toward the Light, to look through the spiritual lens of "higher" and "deeper." Grief births a new self. The spiritual principles of love, connection, compassion, and faith make the painful journey easier and ultimately transcendent.

The shift toward Light, toward spiritual awareness, is your path from suffering to higher healing.

I once spent the night on the side of a mountain in Guatemala, in a tree house overlooking a valley. At 5:00 a.m., the dawn broke and to my surprise, I heard a rousing chorus of hundreds of roosters in the valley all crowing to meet the morning. It was a symphony of sound, a ricocheting rendition of a rooster's acknowledgement of a new day.

This is your new day, the first day of the rest of your life. Remember, all grief stories have a mixture of joy and sorrow. Grief is the story of life. Grief is the story of love. May you savor your love, transform your loss, lift up your consciousness and find peace on your journey, a journey potentially rich with compassion, connection, and faith, but most of all love. The whole point of the journey is love. May you find spiritual comfort, healing, and a life that holds both absence and presence at all times because each is true (and you cannot have one without the other).

Rumi says,

> *Out beyond ideas of wrongdoing and right-doing there is a field. I'll meet you there.*
> *Where the soul lies down in that grass*
> *the world is too full to talk about.*

I would suggest that out beyond ideas of grief and death there is a field. And when the soul lies in that field, life is full again. Feel the grief. Surrender the suffering. Go for the Light-shift.

And so, we end where we began, with the image of a kintsugi bowl, a shattered piece of pottery with gold in its cracks. The expression "go for the gold" is often used to inspire athletes, as in "go for the gold medal." However, as I looked up the expression, I saw that it means more broadly, "attempt to achieve the very best possible outcome." And isn't that what spiritual grief is? Something terrible happened—a life ended, a life shattered. The best possible outcome is to take your pain and transform it into something new, something bigger, something more, something that expands beyond you. That is the spiritual Light in the cracks of grief.

I invite you to move forward, with your loved one in your heart and their love as the wind beneath your wings. Know that your heart can be broken and full simultaneously, luminous between the cracks. Savor the time remaining. Go and greet the day, honoring the Light that will companion you through the darkness.

And together let us share the divine spark of hope.

REFERENCES
AND SUGGESTED READING

Boom, Corrie Ten. *The Hiding Place*. New York, NY: Chosen Books, 2006 (35th Anniversary ed.).

Brach, Tara. *Radical Acceptance*. New York, NY: Bantam, 2004.

Bush, Ashley Davis. *Transcending Loss: Understanding the Lifelong Impact of Grief and How to Make It Meaningful*. New York, NY: Berkley Books, 1997.

———. *Hope and Healing for Transcending Loss: Daily Meditations for Those Who Are Grieving*. New York, NY: Mango Media, 2016.

———. *The Art and Power of Acceptance: Your Guide to Inner Peace*. London, UK: Octopus Publishing, 2018.

———. *The Little Book of Spiritual Bliss*. London, UK: Octopus Publishing, 2020.

Cacciatore, Joanne. *Bearing the Unbearable: Love, Loss, and the Heartbreaking Path of Grief.* New York, NY: Wisdom Publications, 2017.

Devine, Megan. *It's OK That You're Not OK: Meeting Grief and Loss in a Culture That Doesn't Understand.* Boulder, CO: Sounds True, 2017.

Dillard, Sherrie. *I'm Still with You: Communicate, Heal, and Evolve with Your Loved One on the Other Side.* Woodbury, MN: Llewellyn Publications, 2020.

Eden, Donna. *Energy Medicine: Balancing Your Body's Energies for Optimal Health, Joy, and Vitality.* New York, NY: Piatkus Books, 2008.

Frankl, Victor. *Man's Search for Meaning, 4th Edition.* Boston, MA: Beacon Press. 2000.

Frankl, Viktor. *Yes to Life: In Spite of Everything.* Boston, MA: Beacon Press, 2021.

Hanh, Thich Nhat. *No Mud, No Lotus: The Art of Transforming Suffering.* Berkley, CA: Parallax Press, 2014.

Hanson, Chelsea. *The Sudden Loss Survival Guide: Seven Essential Practices for Healing Grief.* Coral Gables, FL: Mango Publishing, 2020.

Hanson, Rick. *Buddha's Brain.* Oakland, CA: New Harbinger Publications, 2009.

Hari, Johann. *Lost Connections: Why You're Depressed and How to Find Hope.* London, UK: Bloomsbury Publishing, 2019.

Ilibagiza, Immaculee (with Steve Erwin). *Left to Tell: Discovering God Amidst the Rwandan Holocaust.* Carlsbad, CA: Hay House, 2006.

———. *Led by Faith: Rising from the Ashes of the Rwandan Genocide*. Carlsbad, CA: Hay House, 2008.

Kessler, David. *Finding Meaning: The Sixth Stage of Grief*. New York, NY: Scribner, 2020.

Li, Qing. *Forest Bathing: How Trees Can Help You Find Health and Happiness*. London, UK: Penguin Life, 2018.

Macpherson, Miranda. *The Way of Grace: The Transforming Power of Ego Relaxation*. Boulder, CO: Sounds True, 2018.

Moorjani, Anita. *Dying to Be Me: My Journey from Cancer, to Near Death, to True Healing*. Carlsbad, CA: Hay House, 2014.

Morter, Sue. *The Energy Codes: The 7-Step System to Awaken Your Spirit, Heal Your Body, and Live Your Best Life*. New York, NY: Atria Books, 2020.

Pittman-Schulz, Kimberley. *Grieving Us: A Field Guide for Living with Loss without Losing Yourself*. Fieldbrook, CA: Kimberley Pittman-Schultz, 2021.

Prevallet, Elaine. *Toward a Spirituality for Global Justice: A Call to Kinship*. Louisville, KY: Sowers Books & Videos, 2005.

Rinpoche, Sogyal. *The Tibetan Book of Living and Dying: The Spiritual Classic and International Bestseller*. San Francisco, CA: HarperSanFrancisco, 2020.

Zuba, Tom. *Permission to Mourn: A New Way to Do Grief*. Rockford, IL: Bish Press, 2014.

GROUP STUDY GUIDE

The following questions are for the purposes of discussing this book and sharing grief experiences in a group setting. I have structured this study guide for a ten meeting format but feel free to organize your book discussion group or grief support group over the number of sessions that best suits the needs of your group.

DISCUSSION QUESTIONS
Week 1—Initial Meeting

1. Allow each person to introduce themselves and to take up to five minutes to share their story of loss(es).
2. What surprises you about the grieving process?
3. What has grief taught you about life and death?

Week 2—Introduction: Light in the Darkness

1. Like a broken bowl, how have you experienced the sharp edges of grief, the feeling of what was once whole now shattered?
2. What does Spirit mean to you? How do you experience that which is greater than self or deep within self?
3. What is it like to imagine a Light-shift in your grief, a moment of feeling supported even in your deep sorrow? Does it feel possible? Impossible? Is there fear? Hope?

Week 3—Part 1. Shock

1. How would you describe your feelings in the first days, weeks, and months after a major loss? Cold? Panicked? Alone? Confused?
2. How did you make it through the impact of shock? What did you find most helpful to survive? What did you do for yourself? How did others help? Is shock still part of your experience?
3. What Light-Shift practice best suits your grief needs? Do tactile experiences shift your feeling state? Do images create an opening to Spirit? Does breath offer a moment of soothing?

Week 4—Part 1. Help!

1. In what ways were you supported and/or misunderstood in the months after your loss?

2. I use the term *Disorganization* to describe "the heart of grief/the bleak midwinter," that lengthy period of time after the shock wears off when your grief is compounded by secondary losses (page 25). What secondary losses did/are you experiencing and how have they affected your grief journey?

3. On page 32, *pain* is defined as the natural agony of losing a loved one, the distress that is grief. *Suffering*, on the other hand, is that additional distress that we experience when we resist or fight the reality of what has happened. Are these concepts helpful for you? How have pain and suffering played out in your path through grief?

Week 5—Part 2. Love

1. Lord Alfred Tennyson wrote, "It is better to have loved and lost than never loved at all," (page 56). How do you feel about this sentiment? Has love been worth the high cost of grief?

2. In what ways has love buoyed you in the ongoing storm of your grief?

3. Forgiveness and acceptance are related but different. Have these concepts played a role in your grief? In what ways do you find it challenging to forgive and accept?

Week 6—Part 2. Connections

1. What is your favorite portal into the natural world? Looking into the sky? Walking in the woods? Swimming in the ocean? Working in your garden? Arranging flowers? Describe a Light-shift that you experienced through your relationship with Nature.

2. On page 77, I list some common ways that people honor their relationship with their deceased loved one. How do you honor your ongoing connection with your loved one? Have you ever experienced a *sign*?

3. How do you understand the term *Higher self* (page 83)? How has your Higher self played a role in your ability to cope with grief?

Week 7—Part 2. Compassion

1. I describe compassion as essentially a spiritual act, as "the ability to understand and sympathize with the painful feelings of others," (page 94). How have you experienced the compassion of others in your own grief?

2. How has your ability to understand and have compassion for other grievers changed since experiencing loss of your own?

3. Being able to have compassion for yourself is essential not only to inner peace but also to being fully compassionate to others. The ACT practice on page 103 describes the three steps to practicing self-compassion. Of the three steps, which is the most challenging and which is the easiest for you?

Week 8—Part 2. Faith

1. *Faith*, a confident belief in that which is unseen, a knowing beyond facts or reason" (page 114). Is this how you see faith? What are other characteristics of faith? How do you know faith when you see it or experience it?

2. What are some examples of how faith has played a role in your life? In your grief?

3. Faith is a personal experience. It is a feeling, a knowing of connection between an inner world and that which is beyond the self. But how does one discern, practice or honor this experience of faith? Can you relate to the Light-shift practices that I offer on page 125? In what ways do you intentionally engage in your faith?

Week 9—Part 3. Transcendence

1. I offer the parable of salt in the lake (page 133) to illustrate the power of an expanded perspective. How is it that the pain of loss can remain the same but begin to feel less painful over time?

2. *Kintsugi*, the Japanese art that turns brokenness into something beautiful, is an important metaphor for transformation through this book. How is it also a symbol for transcendence (making meaning)?

3. Does transcendence feel possible for you in your grief? In what ways big or small have you "extended the reach" of your loved one, used the power of their love to bring meaning into your present world?

Week 10 —Concluding meeting: Reclaiming Life

1. How has your grief restructured and strengthened your "spiritual framework" (page 162)? Is a vertical dimension part of that framework?

2. In what ways has *Light after Loss* helped you to see or experience your grief differently? What Light-shift practice has been most helpful to you?

3. End your final meeting by giving each time

to share their response to this question: What have you most appreciated about this book and sharing your grief experience with others in this group?

ACKNOWLEDGMENTS

To my incredible editor, Rene Sears. I am so grateful for your insightful direction and your generous enthusiasm. To the hardworking team at Viva Editions/Start Publishing, including Meghan Kilduff, Jennifer Do, Ashley Calvano and all others involved in this project, thank you for taking such care in making my vision into a beautiful reality. To Hannah Bennett—thank you for playing an integral part in bringing this book to life at a crucial time in its development.

To my stellar literary agent, John Willig: it is always a pleasure and a delight to acknowledge and thank you. You have been my wizard for over ten years, conjuring book contracts no matter what is going on in the world. You are an author's dream come true and I am ever grateful for your skills, your tenacity, and your support of my work.

To my clients over the years, who have touched me, taught me, and humbled me by sharing their brave journeys: I am in awe of your courage, your strength, and your willingness to grow in spite of tremendous pain.

To my family members and dear friends: I am grateful for your love and ongoing support. Your encouragement and witnessing presence give me strength to follow my call.

To the coronavirus pandemic: while you wreaked havoc around the globe and were responsible for much illness, death, grief, and financial devastation, you have also brought some gifts into our world. You have taught us about isolation and connection, about illness and health, about strength and fragility. And you gave me the time and the inspiration to write this book in 2020 and 2021. May it be a balm to the souls of many. And may we all keep looking for Light-shifts and positive transformations out of tragedy and pain.

With much love to the Brothers of the monastic order of the Society of St. John the Evangelist (SSJE): your steadfast presence has provided me with a hallowed ground of Being for each of my books. And your live-streamed services, an initial response during the global pandemic, was one of the silver linings that kept me connected and inspired during the writing of this book. Blessings upon you.

To Daniel, my beloved best friend, lover, partner,

husband, and soul ballast: once again, you have been the editor and champion to bring another one of my books into the world. I couldn't do it without you. I am forever grateful and honored to have you by my side in this life and beyond.